Near Misses in Cardiac Surgery

Myles Edwin Lee, M.D., FACS
Director
Department of Cardiothoracic Surgery
Centinela Hospital Medical Center
Inglewood, California

Compliments of Bayer Corporation

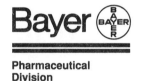

**Pharmaceutical
Division**

Biological Products

Butterworth–Heinemann
Boston   London   Oxford   Singapore   Sydney   Toronto   Wellington

Every effort has been made to ensure that the drug
dosage schedules within this text are accurate and
conform to standards accepted at time of publica-
tion. However, as treatment recommendations
vary in the light of continuing research and clinical
experience, the reader is advised to verify drug
dosage schedules herein with information found
on product information sheets. This is especially
true in cases of new or infrequently used drugs.

 Recognizing the importance of preserving what
has been written, it is the policy of Butterworth–
Heinemann to have the books it publishes printed
on acid-free paper, and we exert our best efforts to
that end.

**Library of Congress Cataloging-in-Publication
Data**
Lee, Myles Edwin.
   Near misses in cardiac surgery/Myles
Edwin Lee.
      p. cm.
   Includes index.
   ISBN 0-7506-9391-6 (pbk. : alk. paper)
   1. Heart–Surgery–Complications–Case studies.
I.   Title.
   [DNLM: 1. Heart Surgery–adverse effects–case
studies. WG 460 L479n]
RD598.L373 1992
617.4'1201–dc20
DNLM/DLC
for Library of Congress   92-49793
                                              CIP

British Library Cataloguing-in-Publication Data
A catalogue record for this book is available from
the British Library.

Butterworth–Heinemann
313 Washington Street
Newton, MA 02158-1626

10 9 8 7 6 5 4 3 2

Printed in the United States of America

You are responsible for the skin and its contents.

Samuel R. Magruder, M.D.
Professor of Anatomy
Tufts University
School of Medicine
Boston, Massachusetts
1961

With affection and respect to Philip N. Sawyer, M.D.
who initiated me into the rites

To the memory of David Preston Boyd, M.D.
who illuminated my path

And with love
to Allison Elizabeth, Evan Preston, and Ladybug
who give relevance to everything that is good
and worth a struggle

Contents

Foreword

Before reading this book, I knew that "Skin and Contents" was the answer I might expect from some surgeon who was asked, "What is your surgical specialty?" However, Dr. Lee makes it clear that "Skin and Contents" is not the punch line to a bad joke (although some people who gave this answer were quite serious), but rather a way to express the need for physicians to look beyond their own specialty and to be aware of not only the whole patient but the whole of medicine. Other principles or messages this book delivers in a most eloquent way are the need for teamwork and the importance of communication, not only among physicians, but among everyone on the healthcare team. Dr. Lee proposes that the eighth deadly sin is Medicine without Teamwork—a sin I have unfortunately seen too many times.

The author readily admits that this book was inspired by his reading *Near Misses in Anesthesia*. He avoids the easy trap of writing a "Look how smart I was to make the diagnosis and save the patient's life" kind of book and instead presents us with a warm, human account based on his great knowledge and experiences. It is my personal belief that teaching with cases of "near misses" is much more effective than a dry discussion of "Complications of . . .".

Besides emphasizing the importance of teamwork and communication, there are other important lessons. The author gives repeated examples of the fact that surgical morbidity and mortality are a function of correct *de*cisions, not *in*cisions. This message should be inscribed on the entrance to every Department of Surgery as well as imprinted on every surgeon. Other valuable lessons include: plan ahead, and don't make the same mistake twice. The key to achieving success is the acquisition of knowledge and its wise, compassionate, and skillful application. Dr. Lee also points out that proper planning and decision-making encompass what must be accomplished, what should be attempted, what is most likely to go wrong, and how to deal with what might go wrong. One of the most important points made in the book concerns the proper question a surgeon or any physician should ask himself, which is "What should be attempted?" and not "What am I capable of doing?" This point is brought home by an example of a patient who suffered because the physician mistakenly asked the latter rather than the former question. This is an example of what we all should have learned in kindergaten—the difference between "can I" and "may I."

Dr. Lee ends the book with his keys to facilitate conversion of experience to effective action. These are *Vigilance* (which is the motto of the American Society of Anesthesiologists), *Communication* (with physicians of the same or a different specialty) that problems exist and must be remedied, a *Standard* approach that emphasizes simplicity and, finally, *Anticipation* of the next step.

This book should be read by surgeons, cardiologist, anethesiologist, and internists. Beyond containing numerous pearls, it is a pleasure to read. Dr. Lee writes exceedingly well, turns graceful phrases, and has a sly wit. Not only will the reader enjoy reading this book but s/he will be in a far better position to prevent a "near miss" from becoming a "direct hit."

Ronald L. Katz, M.D.
Professor of Anesthesiology
Former Chairman, Department of Anesthesiology
Former Chief of Staff, UCLA Medical Center

Preface

Mahatma Gandhi propounded the seven deadly sins to be wealth without work, pleasure without conscience, knowledge without character, commerce without morality, science without humanity, worship without sacrifice, and politics without principle. Without intending to disgrace or trivialize this noble list, I would add an eighth: medicine without teamwork.

The complexity of contemporary medicine has created an age of specialization in which experts master highly distilled bodies of knowledge applicable to one field, virtually to the exclusion of all others. To ensure a consistently successful outcome, however, the delivery of cardiovascular surgical care requires the synthesis of multiple disciplines acting in concert to create a carefully orchestrated sequence of events that, like the notes of a symphony played by a variety of instruments, flow to an inevitable conclusion. It requires teamwork.

Teamwork is the timely and constant exchange of information between disciplines that affects a patient's progress on a moment-to-moment basis. The ability to share effectively one's comments, observations, or demands for immediate action in this manner presupposes that each specialist have at least a basic working knowledge of everyone else's expertise. The anesthesiologist, for example, should be able to assess the validity of a patient's measured hemodynamics by his knowledge and experience blended with observation of the cardiac action in the operative field. The cardiac surgeon should be able to correlate the activity of the heart with the hemodynamics displayed on the monitors. Between them, they should be able to decide if a low blood pressure reading is a function of monitor calibration, air or clot in the arterial line, malposition of the line, a metabolic- or drug-induced lowering of the peripheral vascular resistance, failure of a ventricular septal defect repair, acute malfunction of a prosthetic valve, or ventricular power failure. Furthermore, the physician should not feel embarrassed if an anesthesia technician notices that a stopcock in the arterial line has been partially closed, or if a scrub nurse observes that the abdomen has become noticeably distended as a consequence of the patient's ruptured abdominal aortic aneurysm.

A crucial interdependence exists among the various members of the heart team, making it imperative that they be able to recognize and articulate observations of real or imagined problems that may or may not actually be within the realm of their expertise. The presence of such interaction induces the comfort of shared responsibility, as well as the mutual reassurance and increased likelihood that every consideration in the patient's best interest has been addressed. It is this system of mutual checks and balances that constitutes the essence of team work.

Surgical morbidity and mortality are a direct function of correct *de*cisions, not *in*cisions. The diagnosis of the patient's disease must be correct, the procedure selected for the patient must be correct, and the patient must be correctly selected to withstand the procedure. Although, on occasion, the surgeon must alter a procedure because of unexpected findings or events, the operation is, in general, the most predictable part of the entire diagnostic and therapeutic sequence and is always performed in a standard manner. This must not lull the heart team into the belief that constant vigilance is not necessary. In retrospect, a case that has gone extremely well may regarded as a "slam dunk." During its performance, however, no case can be regarded as "routine."

An illness and its therapy can be as convoluted as a maze. The patient must be *lead* through this maze, not *followed*. Because the patient hasn't a clue where he is going, he will quickly lose his way, choose the path of least resistance, and lead all who follow him into the same bottomless abyss as their white jackets, stethoscopes, strings of clinical pearls, reprints, and best intentions bob helplessly in his wake.

Inspired by Lewis and Fontrier's *Near Misses in Anesthesia* (Butterworth–Heinemann, Boston: 1988), the author presents a similar collection of transiently terrifying dilemmas in this volume of *Near Misses in Cardiac Surgery*, recognized and aborted just in time to prevent irretrievable tragedy. Gathered from institutions in which the author has been a member of the surgical staff, these near-calamities bear witness to the fact that it is not only the patient who goes home with a scar! Having said this, the author, a cardiothoracic surgeon who profited from reading about near misses in anesthesia hopes that not only cardiac surgeons, but anesthesiologists, perfusionists, cardiologists, internists, residents, nurses, technicians, and students will benefit from these truly vexatious experiences.

In order to convey a sense of the pain and anguish endured by members of the team confronting these near-catastrophes, and to challenge the reader to feel that the patient's fate depends upon *his* ability to make the correct decisions quickly, the author has presented cases in the second person, present tense. The cases are, to be sure, anecdotal. Some were approached by methodologies appropriate at the time but not necessarily current. Not all concern matters of technique; some touch upon issues of judgment and decision making in confrontation with complex physiologic, diagnostic, and therapeutic issues. The discussions make no pretense at being exhaustive, and the references provide a mere starting point for further inquiry. The reader should know, however, that all the patients presented here survived the acute situation and that the correct decisions were made sweating it out in the glare of the lights, not in the comfort of an armchair.

Acknowledgments

The author wishes to express his gratitude to Dhun H. Sethna M.D., Director of Cardiac Anesthesia, Cedars Medical Center, Miami, comrade-in-arms and friend, whose thoughtful suggestions greatly improved the scientific and literary content of the manuscript; to Dr. Charles Lee, Professor Emeritus of English and Journalism at the University of Pennsylvania, for his surgical disarticulations and reconstruction of the preface and afterword; to Marilyn Slater, Ph.D., Health Sciences Librarian, Centinela Hospital Medical Center, Inglewood, for her dogged pursuit of the references; to Loussarpi Elizabeth Chahinian, Management Assistant, Department of Cardiothoracic Surgery, Cedars-Sinai Medical Center, Los Angeles, for her resurrection of ancient records; to Paul Nusser, R.N., Cardiovascular Nurse Specialist, Centinela Hospital Medical Center, whose compassion for our patients and their families is legendary; to his colleagues, past and present, who assisted with the management of these patients; to Patricia McLaughlin of LeGwin Associates, Cambridge, Massachusetts, for breaking the code of my hieroglyphic alterations to the manuscript; and to Barbara Murphy, Medical Editor at Butterworth–Heinemann, and her super-staff, who have steadfastly embraced this project from its inception (a forty-five minute transcontinental telephone call from a voice in the wilderness) and delivered the text with dazzling speed from the jungle of tortured syntax into a coherent, reader-friendly format. The author absolves all but himself for errors of omission or commission that may remain in the book.

1

The sun's golden crest is just visible over the mountaintops as you bound out of bed and head for the hospital on an empty freeway enchanted by Chopin's nocturnes. You will operate on a 45-year-old man with an 8-year history of exertional angina. He had exercise-induced anterior segment wall motion abnormalities, a positive exercise thallium study and angiographic confirmation of a long muscle bridge overlying the mid-portion of the left anterior descending coronary artery. Except for some left ventricular apical akinesis, cardiac function was normal. Medical therapy, which included beta blockers and calcium channel blockers, had failed to relieve the symptoms. Dividing a muscle bridge? A resident's case!

At surgery, the aorta was slightly smaller than you expected in a 75 kg patient. You perform the standard cannulations with a 24 French (Fr.) cannula in the ascending aorta, a 51–36 double-caged venous drainage cannula, and an aortic root cardioplegia-venting catheter.

You observe a totally normal bleedback through the aortic cannula and commence cardiopulmonary bypass. At the onset of ventricular fibrillation, you crossclamp the aorta, administer cardioplegia through the aortic root, and begin topical cooling. As you elevate the heart from the pericardium, the back of your right hand encounters a cold, amorphous, posterior mediastinal mass that sends a paralyzing chill to the bottom of your feet. Simultaneously, the perfusionist casually informs you that he cannot maintain a flow rate of more than 1.8 L/min/m² and that the urine output has virtually disappeared. You know what it is but can't believe it is happening to this healthy young patient, the very first from a new referral source, and on such a bright sunny morning.

SOLUTION

Although the ascending aorta appears entirely normal, you quickly open the left mediastinal pleura and confirm your worst fear: an aortic dissection has involved the entire aortic arch and descending thoracic aorta as far as you can palpate. Clamping the venous line, you stop the perfusion, expose the right common femoral artery, and try to cannulate it with a 24 Fr. femoral perfusion catheter. It is too big! Rather than force it in and risk a retrograde dissection as well, you wait for a 22 Fr. and slip it in easily. Clamping the aortic perfusion cannula, you use a scalpel to separate the cannula from the connector and reestablish flow through the femoral line after a quick bleedback to evacuate air.

Reclamping the aorta as close to the innominate artery as possible, you remove the aortic cannula and open the aorta transversely through the cannulation site. This enables you to identify a 1-cm laceration in the posterior wall of the ascending aorta, just where you suspect the tip of the cannula had embedded itself, but find that the laceration lies partially within the jaws of the crossclamp.

While cooling to 15° C, you divide the muscle bridge (which has now become an incidental part of the procedure) and then return to the ascending aorta. You replace the aortic crossclamp between the innominate and left carotid arteries, clamping the innominate artery, as well. This allows full exposure of the laceration, and you deftly close it with four pledgeted sutures. By the time you terminate the procedure, the posterior mediastinal mass is barely palpable, and the patient leaves the operating room in stable condition.

DISCUSSION

The cause of the dissection in this case was the use of a relatively large aortic perfusion cannula with a long, partially curved tip that had, upon insertion and without providing any warning, embedded itself in the posterior wall of a smaller than normal aorta. The brisk jet of blood that exited the tip of the cannula at the onset of cardiopulmonary bypass caused a localized tear in the intima, allowing the dissection to occur.

The incidence of perioperative aortic dissection originating in the ascending aorta is 0.12% but carries a mortality rate of 33% to 62%. The most common etiology is intimal injury caused by a partial occlusion clamp, but dissections have been known to occur at the site of aortic cannulation and at the proximal anastomotic sites of coronary artery bypass grafts.

Perioperative dissections may be avoided by not using partial occlusion clamps, by lowering aortic pressure before any crossclamping or unclamping, and by gentle clamp approximation. It is wise to cannulate the ascending aorta proximally enough so that enough space exists to accomplish exposure and local repair without clamping the brachiocephalic vessels.

An aortic dissection must be considered when there is an unexplained rise in aortic perfusion pressure followed by diminished flow rates and impaired urine output. The diagnosis can be facilitated if the dissection is visible in the ascending aorta, but, as illustrated here, the dissection may not necessarily manifest itself in this manner. The diagnosis in this case was virtually stumbled upon, but the simultaneous combination of the posterior pericardial mass, the perfusionist's complaint, and a high index of suspicion tempered by previous experience led to the patient's survival. Although local repair was possible, more extensive repairs may require aortic replacement with prosthetic grafts.

REFERENCES

1. Kouchoukos NT, Wareing TH: Management of complications of aortic surgery, in Waldhausen JA, Orringer MB, eds. *Complications in Cardiothoracic Surgery* St. Louis, MO: Mosby Year Book, 1991, pages 224–236.
2. Blakeman BM, Pifarre R, Sullivan HJ, Montoya A, Bakhos M, Grieco JG, Foy BK: Perioperative dissection of the ascending aorta: types of repair. J Cardiac Surg 1988:3:9–14.
3. Reig J, Ruiz de Miguel C, Moragas A: Morphometric analysis of myocardial bridges in children with ventricular hypertrophy. Pediatr Cardiol 1990:11:186–190.
4. Nair CK, Dang B, Heintz MH, Sketch MH: Myocardial bridges: effect of propranolol on systolic compression. Can J Cardiol 1986:2:218–221.
5. Furniss SS, Williams DO, McGregor CG: Systolic coronary occlusion due to myocardial bridging—a rare cause of ischaemia. Int J Cardiol 1990:26:116–117.
6. Pey J, de Dios RM, Epeldegui A: Myocardial bridging and hypertrophic cardiomyopathy: relief of ischemia by surgery. Int J Cardiol 1985:8:327–330.

2

A 72-year-old hypertensive patient was admitted because of unstable angina. Cardiac catheterization revealed severe triple vessel coronary artery disease. Prior to the induction of anesthesia, a Swan-Ganz pulmonary artery catheter was advanced to the wedge position through the right internal jugular vein. The right atrial, pulmonary artery, and pulmonary capillary wedge pressures were 10, 33/19, and 15 mm Hg, respectively. After harvesting the saphenous vein, you request the anesthesiologist to administer heparin prior to routine cannulations of the ascending aorta and the right atrium. You are about to begin cardiopulmonary bypass when the anesthesiologist informs you of a torrential tide of red blood that has suddenly flooded the endotracheal tube. You are incredulous! This has arisen at an extremely awkward moment in a heparinized, cannulated patient whose saphenous vein has already been harvested! You must take action now!

SOLUTION

You suspect that the Swan-Ganz catheter has perforated the pulmonary artery, probably on the right side, since most pulmonary artery catheters float to that side. Upon opening the right mediastinal pleura, you identify a diffuse subpleural hemorrhage in the lateral basal segment of the right lower lobe.

You decide to proceed with the operation as planned because of the patient's severe coronary artery disease. You reason that once cardiopulmonary bypass has begun, there should be near-total decompression of the pulmonary circulation with a concomitant reduction in the hemoptysis. Should a pulmonary procedure be required subsequently, it could be performed more safely in a revascularized patient. You complete the coronary artery bypass grafts uneventfully. Prior to separation of the patient from cardiopulmonary bypass, you notice that the right lung has become hyperinflated and perform a bronchoscopy to remove the clot you suspect has obstructed the right main-stem bronchus; thereafter, normal lung dynamics resume. There is no change in the size of the subpleural hematoma, and you terminate bypass. You then start a nitroglycerine drip to reduce preload as the protamine runs in and you are relieved to observe no further bleeding.

DISCUSSION

This patient's hemoptysis resulted from perforation of a peripheral pulmonary artery by a Swan-Ganz catheter. Frequently, this occurs in patients with pulmonary hypertension but can result from miscalculation of the length of catheter required for wedging in an individual patient, as well as from an overzealous technique of insertion. Pulmonary artery perforations can be prevented by using only gentle pressure on insertion. The wedging balloon should always be inflated slowly, with just enough saline introduced to initiate a wedge tracing, and no more. If a patient with pulmonary hypertension must have a pulmonary artery catheter at all, measurements of wedge pressure should probably be avoided. Pulmonary artery catheters should be withdrawn to the main pulmonary artery after the initiation of cardiopulmonary bypass to prevent a hypothermia-stiffened catheter from perforating the pulmonary artery when the heart is elevated from the pericardium for exposure during surgery.

Once catheter-induced hemoptysis has been identified, treatment includes insertion of a double lumen endotracheal tube or an endotracheal tube that incorporates a bronchus blocker, if the bleeding is extensive, to prevent flooding of the opposite main-stem bronchus. Positive end-expiratory pressure may effectively control lesser degrees of bleeding. If these methods fail, lobectomy may be required. If bleeding had continued during the course of the surgery, clamping of the pulmonary hilum would have provided temporary control. Leaving the catheter in place can facilitate direct visualization of the perforation site and permit local control without the necessity of pulmonary resection.

Among other significant problems reported during the insertion of pulmonary artery catheters that require urgent attention is cannulation of the carotid artery with an introducer or sheath. Should this occur in a patient who needs an immediate procedure that requires heparinization, the sheath should be removed and the carotid injury repaired with sutures under direct vision. The induction of right bundle branch block is also a known complication of pulmonary artery catheterization. Should a pulmonary artery catheter be required in a patient with preexistent left bundle branch block, a model with a port for the introduction of a pacing electrode should be employed.

REFERENCES

1. Barash PG, Nardi D, Hammond G, Walker-Smith G, Capuano D, Laks H, Kopriva CJ, Baue AE, Geha AS: Catheter-induced pulmonary artery perforation. Mechanisms, management, and modifications. J Thorac Cardiovasc Surg 1981:82:5–12.
2. Lee ME, Matloff JM, Hackner E: Catheter-induced pulmonary artery hemorrhage (letter to the editor). J Thorac Cardiovasc Surg 1982: 83:796–797.
3. McDaniel DD, Stone JG, Faltas AN, Khambatta HJ, Thys DM, Antunes AM, Bregman D: Catheter-induced pulmonary artery hemorrhage. Diagnosis and management in cardiac operations. J Thorac Cardiovasc Surg 1981:82:1–4.
4. Shah KB, Rao TLK, Laughlin S, et al.: A review of pulmonary artery catheterization in 6245 patients. Anesthesiology 1984:61:271–275.

3

A 65-year-old patient presents with crescendo angina and an eva-
nescent murmur consistent with papillary muscle ischemia. Cardiac catheterization reveals a resting left ventricular end diastolic
pressure of 14 mm Hg, which rises to 43 mm Hg with an episode
of chest pain. This results in 2⁺ to 3⁺ mitral insufficiency. There is
severe triple vessel disease as well, which includes a left main
lesion.

At surgery, the cardiac chambers are of normal size. No thrill
can be palpated in the left atrium even when the blood pressure
is elevated and v waves recorded on the wedge tracing. You decide that repair of the mitral valve is unnecessary and would be
difficult because of the small size of the left atrium. Because of the
inconstant clinical and laboratory findings of mitral insufficiency,
you believe that revascularization alone will suffice. You proceed
with the uneventful bypass of the left anterior descending, diagonal, circumflex, and right coronary arteries with vein grafts. After
appropriate rewarming and evacuation of air from the grafts and
the left ventricle, you terminate cardiopulmonary bypass without
difficulty, although you introduce low dose dobutamine to optimize the hemodynamics. You decannulate the patient, secure
hemostasis, implant pacing wires and mediastinal drains, insert
the sternal wires, and close the incision. The anesthesiologist suddenly informs you that the blood pressure is 50 mm Hg. To your
horror, the regular QRS complexes on the monitor disappear,
and are replaced with unequivocal ventricular fibrillation. You
agonize as to what this could possibly be as you lunge for the
wire cutters.

Upon reentering the chest you find a dilated, cyanotic heart in
full arrest. As you institute open massage, you can't help but notice that the heart has a strange spongy feel, as though it were full
of cellophane. A closer look reveals air bubbles in all the bypass
grafts and coronary arteries as well. You are stunned! The patient
had been decannulated and the chest closed! How could the air
have gotten there?

SOLUTION

You place the patient in the Trendelenburg position, reheparinize, and, with a 14-gauge needle, make multiple fenestrations in all four cardiac chambers, in the aorta and pulmonary artery, and, with a smaller needle, in the grafts. Of considerable interest, no air is present in the ascending aorta beyond the proximal anastomoses of the grafts. You resume cardiac massage as quickly as possible as an assistant cannulates the femoral artery and right atrium. Upon reinstituting cardiopulmonary bypass, you lower the temperature to 28° C, the anesthesiologist administers high-dose steroids and mannitol and induces barbiturate coma with thiopental. After an hour of support, you attempt to terminate bypass. Because of a depressed cardiac output despite the administration of several inotropic agents, you insert an intraaortic balloon through the opposite femoral artery. With the aid of balloon counterpulsation, you are able to not only discontinue the inotropes but find it necessary to place the patient on nitroprusside for control of blood pressure.

In the postoperative period, you maintain the patient at 28° C and continue barbiturate coma for five days. The patient awakens without any neurologic deficit. Despite requiring a tracheostomy and a single hemodialysis for transient renal insufficiency, you discharge the patient a month later without neurologic deficits, able to resume normal activities, including driving a car.

DISCUSSION

During the resuscitation of this patient, an intravenous line used to infuse residual blood from the oxygenator to the patient through the internal jugular vein was noted to have filled with air; the oxygenator was empty. In the absence of a level alarm and automatic pump shut-off, air was pumped into the right heart, causing not only an air lock in the right ventricular outflow tract, and probably through a patent foramen ovale, a massive bolus of air into the left heart and into the ascending aorta as well. The vein grafts, sitting at the highest point of the aorta, siphoned the air into the coronary circulation and stopped the heart, preventing air from entering the brachiocephalic vessels and causing cerebral emboli.

Air embolism can be prevented by compulsive operator attention to the blood level in the oxygenator even with a level detector and automatic pump shut-off, attention to the integrity of the bypass circuitry, and evaluation of all lines for proper direction of flow prior to initiating cardiopulmonary bypass. The surgeon must maintain unswerving adherence to a strict routine for de-airing the cardiac chambers, which includes inversion of the left atrial appendage, ballottement of the heart, and needle venting of the left ventricular apex in all cases. Transesophageal echocardiography can be helpful to assess the presence of significant residual air.

If systemic air embolism occurs during cardiopulmonary bypass, the treatment includes the immediate cessation of arterial perfusion, placement of the patient in the Trendelenburg position, and temporary retroperfusion of the superior vena cava if air is noted in the distal ascending aorta. Induction of hypothermia and barbiturate coma will reduce cerebral metabolism and may limit neurologic injury. Steroids, mannitol, and glycerol may be added to the regimen to reduce cerebral swelling. Hyperbaric oxygenation may be efficacious if transfer to a hyperbaric chamber can be accomplished early after the insult; however, significant resolution of neurologic deficits has been reported even when treatment has begun more than 30 hours following the insult. Transport of an unstable patient to such a facility can be impossible or impractical if the facility is at a great distance.

Other causes of systemic embolization during cardiac surgery include reversal of perfusion or venting lines in the pump heads, detachment of lines, pressurization of non-vented cardiotomy reservoirs or arterial filters, failure to purge air from the venous lines in patients with right-to-left shunts, retained air in the cardiac chambers, aspiration of air through the bone marrow of the divided sternum, aspiration of air into the heart through coronary arteriotomies, retention of air from within a partial occlusion clamp, unexpected resumption of the heartbeat, and faulty techniques while using deep hypothermia and circulatory arrest.

REFERENCES

1. Kurusz M, Wheeldon DR: Risk containment during cardiopulmonary bypass. Seminars in Thorac and Cardiovasc Surg 1990:2:400–409.

2. Mills NL, Morris JM: Air embolism associated with cardiopulmonary bypass, in Waldhausen JA, Orringer MB, eds. *Complications in Cardiothoracic Surgery* St. Louis, MO: Mosby Year Book,1991, pages 60–67.

3. Fundaro P, Santoli C: Massive coronary gas embolism managed by retrograde coronary sinus perfusion. Texas Heart Institute J 1984:11:172–174.

4. Mills NL, Ochsner JL: Massive air embolism during cardiopulmonary bypass: causes, prevention, and management. J Thorac Cardiovasc Surg 1980:80:708–717.

5. Stark J, Hough J: Air in the aorta: treatment by reversed perfusion. Ann Thorac Surg 1986:41:337–338.

6. Robicsek F, Duncan GD: Retrograde air embolism in coronary surgery. J Thorac Cardiovasc Surg 1987:94:110–114.

7. Steward D, Williams WG, Freedom R: Hypothermia in conjunction with hyperbaric oxygenation in the treatment of massive air embolism during cardiopulmonary bypass. Ann Thorac Surg 1977:24:591–593.

8. Armon C, Deschamps C, Adkinson C, Fealy RD, Orzulak TA: Hyperbaric treatment of cerebral air embolism sustained during an open-heart procedure. Mayo Clin Proc 1991:66:565–571.

9. Dunbar EM, Fox R, Watson B, Akrill P: Successful treatment of venous air embolism with hyperbaric oxygen. Postgrad Med J (England) 1990:66:469–470.

4

A 69-year-old patient who had previously undergone a reoperation for coronary artery disease now has recurrent angina 4 months later and requires a third procedure. All his native coronary arteries are closed and, of four vein grafts, only one is patent. Remarkably, left ventricular function is well-preserved. Because of the precarious coronary circulation, you plan to use antegrade-retrograde cardioplegia. The procedure is technically difficult and the targets small. The left internal thoracic artery had been the only graft patent after the patient's first operation but had been injured during the initial reoperation. You graft a lesser saphenous vein to the circumflex and the right internal thoracic artery to the left anterior descending coronary artery. You also graft what you think is the posterior descending coronary artery but discover it to be a coronary vein and ligate the graft. A frustrating case, to be sure, but at least the patient now has three patent conduits.

At the termination of cardiopulmonary bypass, the contractility of the right ventricular free wall remains sluggish despite the administration of amrinone and epinephrine. The cardiac index remains low, and you insert an intra-aortic balloon, which produces stabilization of the hemodynamics and results in a rapidly decreased requirement for pharmacologic support.

After giving protamine, you decannulate the patient. Because of what appears to be a coagulopathy, you begin to administer platelets and fresh frozen plasma. Suddenly, you notice that the QRS pattern on the electrocardiogram has widened and the patient has become hypotensive. This is rapidly followed by a sine-wave pattern, and you find yourself performing open massage on a heart that was entirely stable just moments ago. The heart is not dilated. It is not even fibrillating. It has totally arrested!

SOLUTION

You ask the anesthesiologist if he thinks the patient is having a transfusion reaction or if the patient has received any drug that would account for this. The perfusionist signals for your attention and mentions that the anesthesiologist had corrected a serum potassium of 3.1 meq/L with a slow injection of 20 meq of potassium chloride by syringe. By syringe?

You manage to maintain a blood pressure of 65 to 70 mm Hg systolic with your massage. You order a bolus of epinephrine to tighten the peripheral vasculature and volume expansion to fill the heart. You administer 10 cc of calcium chloride and an ampule of sodium bicarbonate directly into the left ventricle, and request that the anesthesiologist give intravenous insulin and glucose as well. Remarkably, the cardiac action returns and the patient eventually leaves the operating room with stable hemodynamics. He awakens neurologically intact and pursues an uncomplicated course until his release from the hospital.

DISCUSSION

This patient received a cardioplegic dose of potassium at a most inopportune time. The classic sequence of electrocardiographic tracings was apparent and full diastolic arrest with a flaccid heart rapidly ensued. The treatment for potassium toxicity includes the infusion of glucose and insulin, calcium chloride, and sodium bicarbonate, all of which cause potassium to shift to the intracellular position. Hypertonic sodium solutions may be effective as well. None of these measures removes potassium from the body, and a subsequent redistribution of potassium back to the extracellular space must be anticipated. At that time, it may be necessary to administer diuretics and a cation exchange resin, such as sodium polystyrene sulfonate by enema or orally in a 70% sorbitol solution. Intracardiac calcium chloride and bicarbonate were used because the heart was immediately accessible and presented the quickest route for these agents to reach the coronary circulation and perfuse the myocardium.

Certainly, a protamine reaction must be considered in the differential diagnosis of otherwise unexplained postbypass hypotension, especially in a patient who has received protamine on several occasions previously. The rapid administration of protamine produces hypotension by generalized vasodilation, perhaps through histamine or leukotriene release, which causes a reduction in preload and afterload. This response may be exaggerated if the patient is hypovolemic. Protamine does not act as a primary myocardial depressant, however, and does not cause the sequential electrocardiogram changes caused by hyperkalemia. The treatment of a protamine reaction includes circulatory support with epinephrine and, if necessary, reheparinization and the resumption of cardiopulmonary bypass. It is thought that patients who have taken protamine-containing insulin, or who are allergic to shellfish, or who have undergone vasectomy may be especially prone to a protamine reaction.

Protamine may also be responsible for acute pulmonary vasoconstriction with right heart failure and bronchospasm, possibly mediated by thromboxane release induced by heparin-protamine complexes. This is best treated with agents that lower pulmonary vascular resistance, such as isoproterenol (Isuprel), nitroglycerine, or prostaglandin E_1. Cardiac surgical patients with a prior history of exposure to protamine or with any of the risk factors associated with protamine reactions should receive the drug with the aortic and venous cannulas in place to facilitate reinstitution of cardiopulmonary bypass in the event of a protamine reaction.

Other considerations in the patient with sudden unexplained postperfusion hypotension include ABO-incompatible transfusion reactions or an anaphylactic response to drugs such as antibiotics, muscle relaxants, opioids, or colloid volume expanders. Treatment includes cessation of the administration of the antigen, discontinuation of all anesthetic agents, volume expansion, and the administration of epinephrine. Antihistamines and corticosteroids may be given as well.

REFERENCES

1. Levinsky NG: Fluids and electrolytes, in Petersdorf RG, Adams RD, Braunwald E, Isselbacher KJ, Martin JB, Wilson JD, eds. *Harrison's Principles of Internal Medicine*, New York: McGraw-Hill Book Company, 1983, pages 220–230.
2. Hensley FA Jr, Larach DR, Martin DE:

Intraoperative anesthetic complications and their management, in Waldhausen JA, Orringer MB, eds. *Complications in Cardiothoracic Surgery and their Management* St. Louis, MO: Mosby Year Book, 1991, pages 3–19.

3. Horrow JC: Protamine allergy, J Cardiothorac Anesth 1988:2:225–242.

4. Levy JH: The allergic response, in Barash PG, Cullen BF, Stoelting RK, eds. *Clinical Anesthesia* Philadelphia: JB Lippincott Company, 1989, pages 1379–1394.

5. Aren C: Heparin and protamine therapy. Seminars in Thorac and Cardiovasc Surg 1990:2:364–372.

5

Your service hadn't been called to see this patient, but you couldn't help noticing a 56-year-old patient in the intensive care unit sitting bolt upright in bed, sweating, with rapid, labored respirations and a terrified look in his eyes. As politely as possible under the circumstances, you ask his physician, who was writing a lengthy, somewhat leisurely, progress note, what he thought was the matter with this patient. He tells you that the patient had a mitral valve replacement (with a St. Jude prosthesis some years ago) for mitral insufficiency caused by endocarditis. Lost to follow-up, the patient showed up a year later with a left hemiparesis, which subsequently resolved. For the past three weeks, he has complained of dyspnea on exertion. A week prior to his present admission, he was admitted to another institution with congestive heart failure, during which time a Doppler echocardiogram revealed a calculated mitral valve area of 0.9 cm²!

You request permission, because you are just a bit curious, to approach the bedside and discover precisely what you expect: The blood pressure is 90/60, exactly the same as the pulmonary artery pressure, and the pulmonary capillary wedge pressure is 53 mm Hg. There are bilateral rales and no audible valve clicks.

Sometimes there is nothing worse than being right. This patient was being followed when he should have been led. His physician was actually grateful for your studied intrusion into this case and relieved when you told him the patient could be in the operating room in 30 minutes.

SOLUTION

The diagnosis of acute and chronic prosthetic valve thrombosis is obvious and you rush the patient to the operating room, stabilizing the hemodynamics with dopamine. As is routine for all reoperations, you place external defibrillation patches over the right scapula and the apex of the heart. Although you are ready to cannulate the femoral artery and vein, the patient remains stable through the sternotomy. Fortunately, the adhesions are easy to divide and you are able to establish cardiopulmonary bypass uneventfully after exposing the aorta and the right atrium. Because the prosthetic heart valve has old as well as recent thrombus, it is not possible to debride the valve, and you replace it with another St. Jude prosthesis.

DISCUSSION

The mechanism of congestive heart failure in this case is acute thrombosis superimposed upon a chronically-thrombosed prosthetic heart valve that resulted from inadequate anticoagulation. Unless all of the thrombus is relatively recent and the mass of thrombus relatively small, a situation that might permit the use of thrombolytic agents, immediate surgery is mandatory in such cases as a lifesaving measure. The choice of valve re-replacement, biologic versus mechanical, should be made using well-established criteria, modified, perhaps, by the patient's circumstances. If the patient did not understand the importance of anticoagulation but is otherwise compliant and motivated, it is reasonable to use another mechanical prosthesis, especially in the younger patient who would ultimately face a third procedure if a bioprosthesis, known to have limited durability, were employed. In the older patient or one who is known to be noncompliant with prescribed drug regimens, glutaraldehyde-preserved bovine or frozen human valves are excellent substitutes.

Complications from sodium warfarin (Coumadin) therapy should be minimal now that concomitant use of dipyridamole (Persantine) permits lower doses of Coumadin (1.5 times control) with the same effect on limiting thrombosis as regimens calling for higher doses of Coumadin. Problems of over- or underanticoagulation can be avoided by patient education and compulsive follow-up. If Coumadin must be stopped for another surgical procedure, it should be for as short a period as possible. Patients with mechanical valves should be switched over to heparin in these circumstances, as the failure mode of a single tilting disc occluder may result in relatively acute valve stenosis or insufficiency and more rapidly than in patients with bileaflet valves.

In any patient with unexplained or unanticipated congestive heart failure who has had a valve replacement, the immediate and very first task is to assess the function of the prosthesis. This can be accomplished in a few minutes by history, physical examination, and, if time permits, an echocardiogram. No other testing is required. The patient may be stable enough to tolerate general anesthesia with standard cannulations, as in this case, though it is doubtless safer to employ femoral-femoral cannulation as another member of the team enters the chest. In rare instances, cardiopulmonary support may be established percutaneously in the emergency room or in the intensive care unit.

REFERENCES

1. Sawyer PN, Srinivasan S, Lee ME, Martin JG, Murakami T, Stanczewski B: The influence of interface charge on long term function of prosthetic heart valves, in Brewer LA III, ed. *Prosthetic Heart Valves*, Springfield, IL: Charles C. Thomas Publisher, 1969, pages 198–219.
2. Lee ME, Murakami T, Stanczewski B, Parmeggiani A, Srinivasan S, Sawyer PN: Etiology of thrombus formation on prosthetic metal heart valves: the role of spontaneous *in vivo* interfacial potentials and their measurements. J Thorac Cardiovasc Surg 1972;63:809–819.
3. Khan SS, Czer LSC: Antithrombotic therapy after cardiac surgery, in Gray RJ, Matloff JM, eds. *Medical Management of the Cardiac Surgical Patient*, Baltimore: Williams and Wilkins, 1990, pages 221–232.
4. Hellestrand KJ, Morgan JJ, Chang VP: Thrombolytic therapy for a thrombosed Bjork-Shiley tricuspid valve prosthesis. Clin Cardiol 1982;5:347–350.
5. Mattingly WT, O'Connor W, Zeok JV, Todd EP: Thrombotic catastrophe in the patient with multiple Bjork-Shiley prostheses. Ann Thorac Surg 1983;35:253–256.
6. Boskovic D, Elezovic I, Boskovic D, Simin N, Rolovic Z, Josipovic V: Late thrombosis of the

Bjork-Shiley tilting disc valve in the tricuspid position: thrombolytic treatment with streptokinase. J Thorac Cardiovasc Surg 1986:91:1–8.

7. Graver LM, Gelber PM, Tyras DH: The risks and benefits of thrombolytic therapy in acute aortic and mitral prosthetic valve dysfunction: report of a case and review of the literature. Ann Thorac Surg 1988:46:85–88.

8. Baciewicz PA, del Rio C, Goncalves MA, Lattouf OM, Guyton RA, Morris DC: Catastrophic thrombosis of porcine aortic bioprostheses. Ann Thorac Surg 1990:50:817–819.

Lagniappe

When it rains, it pours! You have been asked to see a 38-year-old patient because of shortness of breath. On your initial evaluation she is in congestive heart failure. Two months previously, the patient experienced an embolus to the temporal lobe, documented by a computerized tomographic scan. On the day prior to the current admission, she experienced the sudden onset of cold lower extremities; a saddle embolus was removed by the vascular surgical service using a bifemoral approach. Almost as an afterthought, you are informed by the patient's internist that she had undergone a mitral valve replacement 8 years previously with a Bjork-Shiley prosthesis and that on a recent echocardiogram, not only was there severely impaired motion of the prosthetic disc, but significant echo densities were seen on both sides of the disc, consistent with residual thrombus. Without further delay, you race to the patient's room, stethoscope in hand, to confirm what you already knew would be the case: no valve clicks! You are dumbfounded to learn from the patient *herself* that the valve clicks had disappeared 4 days before admission! No one had told her what that meant. You know what it means. Your plans for the evening have suddenly changed.

6

You have performed uneventful coronary artery bypass grafting in a 73-year-old patient with triple vessel coronary artery disease and normal left ventricular function. During the first six postoperative hours, a liter of blood drains from the chest tubes. Despite vigorous volume replacement, the blood pressure remains 85 mm Hg systolic, with right atrial, pulmonary artery, and pulmonary capillary wedge pressures of 10, 20/13, and 13 mm Hg, respectively. You start a dopamine drip, but the cardiac index rises no higher than 1.83 L/min/m^2, and the patient becomes oliguric. The electrocardiogram is normal, but a repeat chest roentgenogram demonstrates some mediastinal widening with obscuration of the right pulmonary artery, which, previously, had been clearly seen. Physical examination reveals distension of the cervical veins despite the low filling pressures. Right before your eyes, almost defiantly, this patient, with normal biventricular function, is choosing the path of least resistance straight down a black hole from which nothing, not even light, is known to escape, and you are about to follow him unless you can think of something fast!

SOLUTION

Suspicious of pericardial tamponade, although the hemodynamics do not display the usual elevation and equalization of pressures, you return the patient to the operating room where you find that a 10 cm diameter clot has compressed the junction of the superior vena cava and right atrium like a Brobdingnagian fist. Upon removal of the clot, the arterial pressure shoots to 190 mm Hg, requiring control with nitroprusside. A postoperative chest roentgenogram reveals a narrower cardiac silhouette with restored visibility of the right pulmonary artery. The remainder of the patient's course is entirely uneventful.

DISCUSSION

Pericardial tamponade from nonsurgical effusions (uremic, malignant) tend to produce relatively uniform compression of all cardiac chambers. The classically described elevation and equalization of filling pressures in pericardial tamponade requires equal compression of all chambers by a uniformly distributed volume of fluid within the relatively inelastic pericardium. During inspiration, the increased venous return filling the right ventricle limits left ventricular filling, reduces cardiac output, and causes subendocardial ischemia. During expiration, the wedge pressure increases, temporarily enhancing left ventricular filling and cardiac output. This mechanism accounts for the pulsus paradoxus seen with pericardial tamponade.

After cardiac surgery, however, asymmetric compression of a single cardiac chamber may impair cardiac output without the expected hemodynamic pattern. This patient demonstrated an acute superior vena cava syndrome caused by a huge clot that compressed the superior vena cava and restricted flow into the right atrium. Thus, the cervical venous pressure was elevated and the right atrial and pulmonary artery pressures remained within normal limits despite aggressive volume replacement.

Asymmetric, nonuniform single-chamber tamponade is the rule, rather than the exception, following cardiac surgery. The final common pathway of all tamponades is hypotension and depressed cardiac output, but the hemodynamic patterns can have discrete characteristics. For example, right atrial tamponade is characterized by an elevated right atrial pressure in the presence of normal pulmonary artery and pulmonary capillary wedge pressures. It may be necessary to challenge the patient with volume to magnify this difference. Case reports of compression of the pulmonary outflow tract, left atrium, and left ventricle have been described as well.

Technetium-99m ventriculography has been useful in the differentiation of biventricular failure from pericardial tamponade. The presence of radionuclide activity in the pericardial space suggests ongoing bleeding. The diagnosis of pericardial tamponade may be strongly suggested if, at the same time, the radionuclide imaging demonstrates normal biventricular function. More recently, transesophageal echocardiography has proved of value in the diagnosis of right atrial compression following cardiac surgery with greater sensitivity and specificity than transthoracic echocardiography.

The treatment of postoperative pericardial tamponade requires prompt diagnosis and intervention as a lifesaving measure. Early in the postoperative period, it must be anticipated in the patient with unexplained hemodynamic instability and normal ventricular function. It is almost always associated with ongoing bleeding, especially in patients who, once their bleeding has been controlled, form clots that occlude the chest tubes and continue bleeding within the pericardium. Late tamponade occurs usually in patients on anticoagulants and should be suspected in patients who may appear septic or simply are "not doing well."

REFERENCES

1. Lee ME, Gray RJ: Low output states following cardiac surgery, in Gray RJ, Matloff JM, eds. *Medical Management of the Cardiac Surgical Patient*, Baltimore: Williams and Wilkins, 1990, pages 147–151.
2. Hutchins GM, Moore GW: Isolated right atrial tamponade caused by hematoma complicating coronary artery bypass graft surgery. Arch Path Lab Med 1980:104:612–614.
3. Bateman T, Gray R, Chaux A, Lee ME, DeRobertis M, Berman D, Matloff JM: Right atrial tamponade caused by hematoma complicating coronary artery bypass graft surgery: clinical, hemodynamic, and scintigraphic correlates. J Thorac Cardiovasc Surg 1982:84:413–419.

4. Yacoub MH, Cleland WP, Deal CW: Left atrial tamponade. Thorax 1966:21:305–309.
5. Jones MR, Vine DL, Attas M, Todd EP: Late isolated left ventricular tamponade: clinical, hemodynamic, and echocardiographic manifestations of a previously unreported postoperative complication. J Thorac Cardiovasc Surg 1979:77:142–146.
6. Kochar GS, Jacobs LE, Kotler MN: Right atrial compression in postoperative cardiac patients: detection by transesophageal echocardiography. J Am Coll Cardiol 1990:16:511-516.

7

You have been asked for a consultation on an 82-year-old patient 6 days following his admission for a myocardial infarction that was complicated by congestive heart failure and mitral insufficiency. The patient is intubated, on dopamine, with intra-aortic balloon counterpulsation for additional circulatory support. The referring cardiologist, who had signed out to a covering physician for several days, wants you to operate *yesterday*! As you review the chart, however, several things disturb you.

The patient has a low-grade fever. Two cultures from the endotracheal tube grew out *Staphylococcus aureus* and a urine specimen from the Foley catheter grew out greater than 100,000 colonies of *Escherichia coli*. The monitoring lines have not been changed since admission, and the systemic vascular resistance is between 600 and 800 dyne/s/cm^{-5}, lower than one might expect for unloading by balloon counterpulsation alone and raising your suspicion that this elderly patient is septic. The latest chest roentgenogram reveals a pulmonary edema pattern, significantly improved from the admission film, but now with a discrete infiltrate in the right upper lobe. The patient has received no nutritional support, little diuresis, and no antibiotic therapy. Furthermore, you notice that the diagnosis of mitral insufficiency has not been documented by objective means such as an echo Doppler examination, and he has not undergone cardiac catheterization. The referring cardiologist insists you schedule the patient for surgery at once. "At the moment," you mutter to yourself, "this patient doesn't need an operation, he needs a doctor!"

SOLUTION

You notice that after the intra-aortic balloon had been inserted, the pulmonary capillary wedge pressure fell from 60 to 18 mm Hg and the serum creatinine decreased from 4.5 to less than 2 mg/100 mL. In addition, a technetium-99m wall motion study revealed a left ventricular ejection fraction of 60% and a right ventricular ejection fraction of 50%, and the patient has remained hemodynamically stable. Given his favorable hemodynamics, you formulate what some observers perceived to be a daring plan: to effect a metamorphosis of this patient from train wreck to surgical candidate. You hold several discussions with the family, weighing the risks of surgery in an elderly, septic, nutritionally depleted patient versus what might pertain should he be able to withstand a one- to two-week delay to correct these conditions. Your recommendation is that only after this has been accomplished should the patient undergo cardiac catheterization. You win the confidence of the patient's family who appreciate your concern and candor.

Over the next 2 weeks, you accomplish what even *you* weren't certain could be done. You begin total parenteral nutrition, aggressive diuresis, and appropriate antibiotics. Slowly, you wean the patient from dopamine, remove the intra-aortic balloon, and extubate him. Before long, you transfer him from the intensive care unit to the step-down unit where, over a period of days, the patient actually becomes ambulatory. Following the extraction of several infected teeth, you signal the cardiologist that the patient is ready for catheterization. This reveals subtotal obstruction of the left anterior descending and circumflex coronary arteries and a 60% narrowing in the proximal third of the right coronary artery. There is 4+ mitral regurgitation but not across a broad front.

At surgery, there is no transmural infarction. The left atrium is small. The mitral valve reveals rupture of a small, infarcted papillary muscle, suggesting, as did the patient's clinical course, that volumetrically, the regurgitant jet was 4+ more on the basis of extent into the atrium rather than on the basis of its breadth across the valve. Surgery includes vein grafts to the left anterior descending, circumflex, and right coronary arteries, as well as mitral valve replacement with a porcine bioprosthesis. The patient remains alive and well five years later.

DISCUSSION

This case illustrates dramatically that *de*cisions impact surgical morbidity and mortality more than *in*cisions. Whereas the incision is always the same, the decisions leading to it must include an intensive determination of the cardiac as well as the noncardiac risks. With a left ventricular ejection fraction of 60%, no prior myocardial infarction, good coronary targets, absence of hepatic dysfunction, and manageable hemodynamics despite new onset mitral insufficiency, this patient's risk of surgery, strictly from the cardiac viewpoint, was low. However, to have proceeded with an emergency operation in an infected, malnourished octogenarian invited the risk of disastrous septic complications, including exacerbation of his pneumonia, wound infections, and gram-negative sepsis with its sequellae. Any surgical procedure performed as an emergency and under such circumstances triples the risk of operative mortality and, should the patient survive long enough, results in a cascade of complications that are predictable and, therefore, preventable.

The management of this case was as much art as science. It was by no means a certainty that this patient would survive his 2-week period of rehabilitation, but once he did, his primary risk factors were his age and the limitations of functional reserve dictated by his age on organs other than the heart. The surgeon, in circumstances such as these, must deal not only with the impact of surgery on the patient but also with the emotional strain placed on the family should an ill-timed operation lead to multisystem complications that result in a mortality after a 3-month stay in the intensive care unit. To accomplish this goal, the surgeon must tactfully, yet forcefully, defend his prerogative that patient selection and the timing of surgery are justifiable as determinants of patient survival, and are just as important as the mechanics of a well-performed operation.

REFERENCES

1. Naunheim KS, Kern MJ, McBride LR, et al.: Coronary artery bypass surgery in patients aged 80 years and older. Am J Cardiol 1987:59:804-807.
2. Naunheim KS, Fiore AC, Wadley JJ, McBride LR, Kanter KR, Pennington G, Barner HB, Kaiser GC, Willman VL: The changing profile of the patient undergoing coronary artery bypass surgery. J Am Coll Cardiol 1988:11:494–498.
3. Grover FL, Hammermeister KE, Burchfiel C, et al.: Initial report of the veterans administration preoperative risk assessment study for cardiac surgery. Ann Thorac Surg 1990:50:12–28.
4. Teoh KH, Christakis GT, Weisel RD, Katz AM, Tong CP, Mickleborough LL, Scully HE, Baird RJ, Goldman BS: Increased risk of urgent revascularization. J Thorac Cardiovasc Surg 1987:93:291–299.
5. Scott, WC, Miller DC, Haverich A, Mitchell RS, Oyer PE, Stinson EB, Jamieson SW, Baldwin JC, Shumway NE: Operative risk of mitral valve replacement: discriminant analysis of 1329 procedures. Circulation 1985:72 (Suppl. II), II–108.
6. Czer LSC, Gray RJ, DeRobertis MA, Bateman TM, Stewart ME, Chaux A, Matloff JM: Mitral valve replacement: impact of coronary artery disease and determinants of prognosis after revascularization. Circulation 1984: 70 (Suppl. I): I–198–207.

8

A 52-year-old patient with no prior cardiac history was admitted to a community hospital with chest pain that was associated with a rise in creatine phosphokinase of 1300 international units, but with no electrocardiographic changes. Two days later, a low level treadmill test results in precordial ST-segment depression but no chest pain. Shortly after the treadmill test, the patient experiences recurrent chest pain associated with precordial ST-segment elevation and receives a tissue plasminogen activator for thrombolysis of what is presumed to be obstruction of the left anterior descending coronary artery. He is then transferred to the catheterization laboratory in cardiogenic shock where an intra-aortic balloon is inserted. With intra-aortic balloon counterpulsation, the cardiac output is 2.6 L/min with a heart rate of 130 and a stroke volume of 20 cc.

Coronary angiography reveals flush occlusion of the left anterior descending, absence of major circumflex branches, and minor irregularities in the right coronary artery. Although a guide wire passes through the left anterior descending lesion and the cardiologist makes multiple attempts at percutaneous transluminal coronary angioplasty, there is no angiographically apparent perfusion into the left anterior descending artery. The patient is now 8 hours into his infarction and deteriorating. The cardiologist desperately asks if you can bypass the left anterior descending.

SOLUTION

You explain to the cardiologist that under these circumstances the operative mortality with conventional bypass surgery approaches 100%. Furthermore, even if a graft were constructed to the left anterior descending, it would very likely not perfuse the anterior wall because of the no-reflow phenomenon. You urge the cardiologist and the patient's family to transfer the patient to a university center for what you believe to be the patient's only chance: insertion of a left ventricular assist device and subsequent cardiac transplantation. Although the patient requires endotracheal intubation just before being placed in the ambulance, the transfer is successful.

In the operating room, ventricular fibrillation occurs concurrent with the sternotomy, and cannulation is accomplished during the performance of open cardiac massage. The anterior wall is edematous and cyanotic. A vein graft to the left anterior descending is constructed, but the patient cannot be separated from bypass, despite the employment of controlled reperfusion with glutamate-aspartate enriched cardioplegia. He is placed on a centrifugal left ventricular assist device, which sustains him for 4 days. At that time, a donor heart is located and the patient is successfully transplanted. He leaves the hospital in 9 days and remains well 4 years later.

DISCUSSION

Myocardial reperfusion is more complicated a matter than simply the quick restoratione of blood flow through an obstructed artery. Numerous investigators have demonstrated that oxygen-derived free radicals are significant contributors to the cellular and subcellular disruption associated with ischemia and reperfusion. This results in myocyte dysfunction as well as the vascular endothelial swelling which causes the no-reflow phenomenon. Therapeutic interventions to prevent or control the extent of free radical formation such as leukocyte depletion during cardiopulmonary bypass, lidocaine inhibition of leukocyte activation, inhibition of superoxide production by the xanthine oxidase inhibitor allopurinol, and inhibition of the iron-catalyzed break down of hydrogen peroxide to hydroxyl ions, have all received intense laboratory and clinical scrutiny. Free radical scavengers such as superoxide dismutase, catalase, peroxidase, and reduced glutathione have also been studied.

This patient had ongoing ischemia over a 2-day period that resulted in infarction and cardiogenic shock of 8 hours duration. The patient's ventriculogram suggested that significant myocardial edema was present. The extent of myocardial edema has been shown to correlate directly with the activation of granulocytes in an ischemic segment. Although reperfusion with agranulocytic blood has been shown to limit the amount of edema in such segments, attenuate the no-reflow phenomenon, and limit infarct size, it was likely that, under the given circumstances, any attempt at emergency revascularization alone was at significant risk of failure, and that advanced methods of circulatory assist and, ultimately, cardiac transplantation had to be available.

The most frequent indications for mechanical circulatory assist include ventricular power failure following cardiac surgery, cardiogenic shock as a consequence of myocardial infarction, and acute rejection of the transplanted heart. About 70% of such situations can be salvaged with pharmacologic support and intra-aortic balloon counter-pulsation. Should the patient remain hypotensive with a cardiac index of less than 1.8 L/min/m^2 and a pulmonary capillary wedge pressure of greater than 25 mm Hg, then direct ventricular support with uni- or bi-ventricular assist devices is indicated.

As summarized in the report by Miller, who reviewed the efficacy of ventricular assist devices in 451 postcardiotomy cardiogenic shock patients between 1978 and 1988, 45% could be weaned from left and right ventricular assist devices, but only 24% of the patients were ultimately discharged from the hospital, irrespective of the type of assist device used and whether one or both ventricles were supported. The discharged patients experienced a 2-year survival of 88% in New York Heart Association (NYHA) class I or II if the 30-day mortality patients were eliminated from the statistics, and 47% if they were not.

Long-term survival rates improve significantly if ventricular assist devices are used as bridges to transplantation in patients who otherwise are candidates for transplantation, but who develop refractory cardiogenic shock before a suitable donor heart can be obtained. In a series of 184 such patients supported by a variety of pumps reviewed by Hill, 130 patients (70%) underwent cardiac transplantation, of which 85 patients (46%) were discharged from the hospital. The results are twice as good compared to Miller's group of patients, in which transplantation was not performed. Compared with elective transplantation, where the 1-, 5-, and 10-year survivals in a combined series of 6500 patients are now 90%, 85%, and 72%, respectively, the results of transplantation in patients who have received ventricular assist devices as a bridge to transplantation reflect learning curves with the various devices and the factors that always complicate the course of such patients: multisystem organ failure, hemorrhagic complications, and infection.

REFERENCES

1. Allen BS, Buckberg GD, Fontan FM, Kirsh MM, Popoff G, Beyersdorf F, Fabiani J-N, Acar C: Superiority of surgical reperfusion vs PTCA in Acute Coronary Occlusion. Presented at the 72nd Annual Meeting of the Association for Thoracic Surgery, Los Angeles, CA, 27 April, 1992.

2. Jeremy RW, Links JM, and Becker LC: Progressive failure of coronary flow during reperfusion of myocardial infarction: documentation of the no reflow phenomenon with positron emission tomography. J Am Coll Cardiol 1990:16:695–704

3. Royston D: Blood cell activation. Seminars in Thorac and Cardiovasc Surg 1990:2:341-357.

4. Colman RW: Platelet and neutrophil activation in cardiopulmonary bypass. Ann Thorac Surg 1990:49:32–34.

5. Menasché P, Piwnica A: Free radicals and myocardial protection: a surgical viewpoint. Ann. Thorac Surg 1989:47:939–945.

6. Lee ME: Mechanical support of the circulation, in Gray RJ, Matloff JM, eds. *Medical Management of the Cardiac Surgical Patient.* Baltimore: Williams and Wilkins, 1991, pages 164–173.

7. Miller CA, Pae WE Jr, Pierce WS: Combined registry for the clinical use of mechanical ventricular assist devices: post-cardiotomy cardiogenic shock. Trans Am Soc Artif Int Org 1990:36: 43–46.

8. Hill JD: Bridging to cardiac transplantation: Ann Thorac Surg 1989:47:167–171.

9. Lower RR, Shumway NE: Studies on the orthotopic homotransplantation of the canine heart. Surg Forum 1960:11:18.

10. Fragomeni LS, Kaye M: The registry of the international society for heart transplantation: fifth official report. J Heart Transplantation 1988:7:249–253.

9

A 51-year-old patient presents with the acute onset of precordial chest pain radiating to the neck and back. The electrocardiogram is normal and there is no enzyme rise. He had undergone coronary artery bypass grafting to the left anterior descending and first and second circumflex coronary arteries 10 years previously. At that time his ascending aorta was enlarged. A computerized tomographic scan of the chest on this admission reveals an aortic dissection involving the aortic root. Cardiac catheterization reveals total obstruction of the native coronary circulation. There is a 75% narrowing of the left anterior descending graft, a normal first circumflex graft, and total obstruction of the second circumflex graft. Although he is currently asymptomatic, you know this patient needs urgent replacement of the ascending aorta, aortic valve replacement or resuspension, and myocardial revascularization. When you examine him, however, you are dismayed to find a draining sinus tract in the lower part of the sternotomy incision. The patient says it has been there ever since his initial operation.

SOLUTION

Since the patient remains stable, you elect to perform a sinogram, which reveals a tract leading to the lowest wire in the sternotomy incision. There is no evidence of osteomyelitis on this study or on the computerized tomographic scan.

Under general anesthesia and with an arterial line to permit precise control of the heart rate and blood pressure, you remove the lowest three sternal wires and excise the sinus tract. The patient remains in the intensive care unit, sedated, at strict bed rest, on nitroprusside and a beta blocker, with frequent debridement and dressing changes. Cultures from the sinus tract grow out a species of *Serratia,* and you add an aminogly-coside to the patient's antibiotic regimen. Twelve days after initiating this therapy, the patient experiences recurrent precordial chest pain. A prominent murmur consistent with aortic insufficiency appears for the first time. As you take the patient to the operating room, you can only hope that by now the sternal incision has been sterilized.

After cannulation of the femoral artery and vein, you carefully enter the anterior mediastinum without injuring the ascending aorta, cannulate the right atrium, and begin cardiopulmonary bypass. After cooling to 24° C, you crossclamp the ascending aorta and open it. You administer cardioplegia directly through the ostia of the left anterior descending and first circumflex grafts and then place new grafts in the postero-lateral branch of the right, the left anterior descending, and the second circumflex coronary arteries with sequential infusion of cardioplegia into each graft at its completion.

The aortic dissection, as anticipated, has originated in the aortic root. You replace the aortic valve and ascending aorta with a valved conduit constructed at the operating table from a bileaflet mechanical valve and a collagen-coated Dacron graft. You then ligate the coronary ostia, suture the vein grafts to the aortic graft prosthesis, and perform the distal aortic anastomosis. Termination of cardiopulmonary bypass necessitates intra-aortic balloon pumping for hemodynamic stability. The patient survives in excess of five years with no incisional or systemic infection.

DISCUSSION

This patient had been seen initially at another institution and actually had been sent home after his computerized tomographic scan and coronary arteriogram; the consulting surgeon had declined to operate because of the draining sinus tract. Once transferred to a tertiary care center, the decision-making process included consideration of immediate surgery, which carried a significant risk of systemic and local infection, as opposed to an attempt to cure the sinus tract first under controlled circumstances. The latter course was pursued, with surgery precipitated by the development of heart failure secondary to the risk of acute aortic insufficiency. It was fortunate that enough time had elapsed to allow cure of the sternal infection.

Among the technical difficulties presented by this patient, in addition to the risk of aortic disruption during sternotomy, was the difficulty of myocardial protection in the presence of totally obstructed native coronary arteries and arteriosclerotic vein grafts, one of which was completely occluded. As evidenced by the need for intra-aortic balloon counter-pulsation, myocardial protection was not optimal, even though cardioplegia had been infused into the grafts. The addition of retrograde cardioplegia would have resulted in more uniform myocardial cooling. External defibrillation pads should have been placed over the right scapula and the apex of the left ventricle to allow cardioversion should ventricular fibrillation have occurred before or during sternotomy and the dissection of the anterior mediastinum.

Acute dissection of the ascending aorta is a surgical emergency that requires immediate intervention to prevent complications such as aortic rupture, pericardial tamponade, coronary occlusion, and aortic insufficiency. Since this patient had undergone prior cardiac surgery and already had total occlusion of his native coronary arteries, and with adhesions already obliterating the pericardial space, the occurrence of the first three of these complications was considered unlikely; indeed, acute aortic insufficiency precipitated surgery.

Patients frequently present vexing combinations of problems. The successful resolution of cases such as this one depends upon the physician's ability to weigh the risks and benefits of different courses of action, an ability that is built upon a foundation of textbook knowledge, but is nurtured by years of experience.

REFERENCES

1. Bentall H, DeBono A: A technique for complete replacement of the ascending aorta. Thorax 1968:23:338–339.
2. Kouchoukos NT, Marshall WG Jr, Wedige-Stecher TA: Eleven-year experience with composite graft replacement of the ascending aorta and aortic valve. J Thorac Cardiovasc Surg 1986:92:691–705.
3. Cabrol C, Gandjbakhc I, Pavie A: Surgical treatment of ascending aortic pathology. J Cardiac Surg 1988:3:167–180.
4. Crawford ES, Svensson LG, Coselli JS, Safi HJ, Hess KR: Surgical treatment of aneurysm and/or dissection of the ascending aorta, transverse aortic arch, and ascending aorta and transverse aortic arch: factors influencing survival in 717 patients. J Thorac Cardiovasc Surg 1989:98:659–674.
5. Lewis CTP, Cooley DA, Talledo O, Murphy MC: Experience with surgical repair of aortic root aneurysms: results in 280 patients. (abstract). Presented at the Society of Thoracic Surgeons 27th annual meeting 18–20 February 1991.

10

A 49-year-old patient with a long history of a heart murmur presents with the recent onset of progressive exercise intolerance. Doppler echocardiography reveals significant aortic insufficiency and pronounced ventricular dilation. Cardiac catheterization reveals normal coronary arteries. You recommend aortic valve replacement because of the progression in symptoms and the enlarged ventricle.

At surgery, you cannulate the ascending aorta, the right atrium with a two-stage venous cannula, and place a vent through the right superior pulmonary vein into the left ventricle. You begin cardiopulmonary bypass with the left ventricular vent activated to prevent overdistension of the left ventricle. At the onset of ventricular fibrillation, you crossclamp the aorta and introduce crystalloid cardioplegia by direct cannulation of each coronary ostium, and provide topical cooling with cold saline as well. After excising the diseased aortic valve, you irrigate the cavity of the left ventricle with cold saline, implant a bileaflet mechanical prosthesis, and close the aorta. You complete rewarming and de-airing in a routine manner and terminate cardiopulmonary bypass. Nothing to it!

Shortly after you remove the aortic cannula, however, ventricular fibrillation occurs, which is refractory to multiple attempts at defibrillation.

SOLUTION

As you perform cardiac massage, your assistant recannulates the ascending aorta and you resume cardiopulmonary bypass. Once you have manually decompressed the left ventricle, you are able to convert it to a regular rhythm with a single countershock. You notice at this time that the anterior segment of the left ventricle is significantly hypocontractile and that the pulmonary artery diastolic pressure rises acutely when you attempt to separate the patient from bypass. You give the patient a loading dose of Amrinone (a phosphodiesterase inhibitor) and start an epinephrine drip. In addition, you insert an intra-aortic balloon and observe the patient for another 45 min before successfully terminating cardiopulmonary bypass. The patient now has a cardiac output of 7 L/min with somewhat improved left ventricular contractility. The remainder of the patient's course is uneventful and he remains symptomatically improved 3 years later.

DISCUSSION

Postoperative left ventricular power failure has numerous etiologies. Patients who enter cardiac surgery with impaired left ventricular function are at higher risk of operative cardiac mortality. Impaired ventricular function may result from myocardial infarction, myocardial ischemia, or alterations of the geometry of ventricular contractility caused by myocardial dilation or hypertrophy secondary to mechanical abnormalities such as valvular stenosis or insufficiency, ventricular aneurysm, ventricular septal defects, or recurrent episodes of supraventricular tachycardia.

Ventricular dysfunction may occur intraoperatively as well and result from inadequate myocardial protection, air embolism, incomplete revascularization, or technical problems relating to specific procedures. The difficulties encountered in the present case probably resulted from an uneven delivery of cardioplegia into the coronary system. Direct coronary perfusion was employed using self-sealing cannuli. While it is possible that an inadequate amount of cardioplegia was delivered to the myocardium in total, it is also possible that the tip of the left coronary cannula was directed so as to exclude the left anterior descending territory from much of the flow, with preferential flow into the circumflex coronary artery. Early documentation of inadequate cardioplegia delivery to the left anterior descending territory could have been provided by measurement of the interventricular septal temperature.

The advent of retrograde cardioplegia permits more uniform delivery of cardioplegic solutions throughout the myocardium, especially in the presence of multiple coronary obstructions or in patients with thickened or dilated ventricles. Under these circumstances, cardioplegia delivered antegrade will seek the path of least resistance into the least-obstructed coronary arteries. This may result in myocardial segments subtended by the most obstructed arteries remaining relatively warm with ongoing localized electrical activity that has been associated with the development of intramyocardial cellular acidosis, high energy phosphate depletion, and ultimate cellular dysfunction. Retrograde cardioplegia, administered through the coronary sinus or into the right atrium, will more uniformly perfuse and cool the myocardium. If given in the right atrium, with bicaval cannulation and compression of the pulmonary artery, cardioplegia will enter not only the coronary sinus but the thebesian veins as well; in addition, there will be direct endocardial cooling of the right atrium and the right ventricle. Retrograde cardioplegia, in conjunction with antegrade cardioplegia, should eliminate the need for direct coronary artery cannulation and its inherent risks of misdirected flow and local intimal trauma, which has been responsible for late coronary ostial stenoses. It should also eliminate the need for the administration of cardioplegic solutions through vein grafts thus avoiding the potentially damaging effects of potassium-containing solutions on the venous endothelium.

Newer types of cardioplegic solutions include preparations designed to be administered continuously at normothermia in either antegrade or retrograde fashion with nutrients designed to enable myocardial cellular resuscitation during the course of surgery. The safety of this method remains to be proved by multicenter studies.

REFERENCES

1. Menasché P, Subayi J-B, Piwnica A: Retrograde coronary sinus cardioplegia for aortic valve operations: a clinical report on 500 patients. Ann Thorac Surg 1990:49:556–564.
2. Menasché P, Subayi J-B, Veyssie L, Le Dref O, Chevret S, and Piwnica A: Efficacy of coronary sinus cardioplegia in patients with complete coronary artery occlusions. Ann Thorac Surg 1991:51:418–423.
3. Mankad PS, Chester AH, Yacoub MH: Role of potassium concentration in cardioplegic solutions in mediating endothelial damage. Ann Thorac Surg 1991:51:89–93.
4. Yates JD, Kirsh MM, Sodeman TM, et al.: Coronary ostial stenosis: a complication of aortic valve replacement. Circulation 1974:49:530–534.
5. Salerno TA, Houck JP, Barrozo CAM, Panos A, Christakis GT, Abel JG, Lichtenstein SV: Retrograde continuous warm blood cardioplegia: a new concept in myocardial protection. Ann Thorac Surg 1991:51:245–247.

11

A 70-year-old patient suffers an anterolateral myocardial infarction following a total knee replacement. Subsequent cardiac catheterization reveals akinesis of the anterolateral and apical portions of the left ventricle. There are vigorous contractions of the base of the heart and no mitral insufficiency. The left anterior descending coronary artery is totally obstructed without collateralization, and the circumflex and right coronary arteries are normal.

One month later the patient experiences shortness of breath. A workup for pulmonary embolization, which includes pulmonary angiography, is negative. The patient is treated medically for congestive heart failure over the course of a month in the hospital, without improvement. During this time the patient is virtually bedridden, with the effort of rising from bed to sit in a chair leaving him gasping for breath.

At this point, you see the patient in consultation. The patient's blood pressure is 109/73 mm Hg, pulse 96, and respirations 20. There are cervical venous distensions halfway to the angle of the jaw and bibasilar rales. The point of maximum impulse is diffuse in the fifth intercostal space. At your recommendation, cardiac catheterization is repeated, revealing a right atrial pressure of 6, a right ventricular pressure of 54/10, a pulmonary artery pressure of 57/25, and a pulmonary capillary wedge pressure of 27 mm Hg. The coronary arteries are unchanged, and there is no mitral insufficiency; however, there had been a significant increase in the size of the aneurysm and decreased contractility of the base of the heart. The patient and his family await your recommendation.

SOLUTION

You decide that there are enough clinical and laboratory data to explain this patient's continuing deterioration on the basis of an altered geometry of left ventricular ejection resulting in progressive congestive heart failure. You decide to resect the ventricular aneurysm and reconstruct the ventricle so that the mechanics of ventricular ejection return as close to normal as possible.

At surgery, you encounter an extremely large anterolateral and apical aneurysm filled with a laminated clot that occupies the apex and anterior segments and extends along the septum toward the left ventricular outflow tract, raising the possibility that the left ventricular outflow tract was partially obstructed by the clot. As anticipated, the anterior part of the septum is thinned out and aneurysmal as well.

You place multiple pledgeted sutures through the redundant infarcted septum and bring them out through the para-septal left ventricular wall. Once tied, these sutures eliminate the redundancy in the septal tissue in a manner analogous to taking a reef in the mainsail of an ocean-going sloop. You place two polypropylene purse-string sutures around the circumference of the aneurysm at the junction of normal and scarred tissue and tighten them so that the residual defect is 4 to 5 cm in diameter, and then implant a collagen-coated Dacron patch to recreate the ventricular apex, finally covering the apex with residual aneurysm tissue.

After having been in the hospital for about 5 weeks preoperatively, the patient leaves the hospital in 8 days after an uneventful post-operative course, without any further episodes of congestive heart failure, and has remained symptom-free for a year.

DISCUSSION

This patient languished in the hospital for over a month before cardiac surgical consultation was obtained. The repeat catheterization provided dramatic documentation of the progressive deterioration in ventricular function that had occurred in a 2-month period.

The common indications for resection of a ventricular aneurysm include systemic embolization, ventricular arrhythmias, and congestive heart failure refractory to medical therapy. The genesis of congestive heart failure associated with a ventricular aneurysm is complex. The aneurysm itself can become so large as to collect a significant volume of blood during diastole. During systole, when the aneurysm exhibits paradoxical motion, the blood it contains swirls about in the aneurysm rather than being ejected into the systemic circulation, creating the hemodynamic equivalent of functional mitral insufficiency. As the aneurysm enlarges further, the residual contracting elements of the left ventricle are both stretched and splayed apart by the ring of tissue forming the junction of normal and infarcted muscle, which impairs the ability of these segments to contribute effectively to left ventricular emptying. This distorted geometry of contraction may also result in altered vectors of contraction of the papillary muscles of the mitral valve, causing mitral insufficiency.

Other causes of impaired ejection in left ventricular aneurysm include obstruction by clot of the left ventricular outflow tract, as observed in this case, and impairment of right ventricular filling by an aneurysm so large that it virtually results in an auto-tamponade.

The traditional technique of ventricular aneurysm resection includes removal of aneurysmal tissue and closure of the resultant defect using a straight, pledget-reinforced suture line that essentially amputates the apex of the heart. The technique employed in this case, described by Jatene and modified by McGiffin, attempts to restore the ventricular cavity to a normal shape and to thereby optimize the dynamics of left ventricular emptying by restoring normal vectors of contraction. Whether this will prove better over the long term compared to the amputation method remains to be seen.

REFERENCES

1. Cooley DA, Hallman GL, Henly WS: Left ventricular aneurysm due to myocardial infarction: experience with 37 patients undergoing aneurysmectomy. Arch Surg 1964:88:114–121.
2. Cohen M, Packer M, Gorlin R: Indications for left ventricular aneurysmectomy. Circulation 1983:67:712–722.
3. McGiffin DC, Kirklin JK: Patch repair of the left ventricular free wall following aneurysmectomy. Ann Thorac Surg 1987:43:441–442.
4. Jatene AD: Left ventricular aneurysmectomy: resection or reconstruction? J Thorac Cardiovasc Surg 1985:89:321–331.
5. Komeda M, David T, Malik A, Ivanov J, Sun Z: Operative risks and long-term results of operation for left ventricular aneurysm. Ann Thorac Surg 1992:53:22–29.

12

A 67-year-old patient presents with the recent onset of angina pectoris associated with a positive treadmill test. Cardiac catheterization reveals a 90% obstruction in the proximal left anterior descending and an 80% obstruction in the proximal portion of the right posterior descending coronary artery. The cardiologist decides to perform percutaneous transluminal coronary angioplasty of the left anterior descending. Although there is evidence of a localized dissection at the site of angioplasty in the left anterior descending, the lesion appears less restrictive than before the procedure, and it is declared a success. During the night, however, the patient experiences mild angina. Repeat angiography the next morning reveals persistence of the dissection and a recurrent subtotal obstruction at the angioplasty site. Another attempt at angioplasty of the left anterior descending not only fails to open the left anterior descending but results in a clot that causes subtotal obstruction of the circumflex coronary artery as well. The cardiologist inserts a bailout catheter into the left anterior descending and calls you for an emergency cardiac surgical consultation.

SOLUTION

Despite having an acute left main equivalent lesion, enough flow perfuses the left coronary branches to allow the patient's hemodynamics to remain stable during the precipitous transfer to a hastily prepared operating room (fortunately, one was available). At surgery, you notice some epicardial hemorrhage over the proximal portion of the left anterior descending. Remarkably, there is normal left ventricular contractility with no evidence of transmural myocardial infarction. Once on cardiopulmonary bypass, you administer cardioplegia through the aortic root and directly through the arteriotomies in the left anterior descending and circumflex coronary arteries. In the interest of performing an expeditious procedure under adverse circumstances, you forgo a dissection of the left internal thoracic artery and construct saphenous vein grafts to the left anterior descending, circumflex, and right posterior descending coronary arteries. The patient makes an uneventful recovery and remains well over 4 years later.

DISCUSSION

The advent of coronary balloon angioplasty and other interventions, such as atherectomy, roto-ablation, and laser angioplasty, have enabled cardiologists to participate in the treatment of coronary artery disease as well as in its diagnosis. It is important that, in each case, the risk of angioplasty failure be weighed against the risk of elective coronary artery bypass grafting, and against the risk of emergency coronary artery bypass grafting in patients experiencing a myocardial infarction with or without cardiogenic shock. A cumulative summary of 15 series of patients, reviewed by Parsonnet et al., revealed an 18.8% operative mortality rate for coronary artery bypass grafting after failed angioplasty compared to a 1.5% operative mortality rate for elective coronary artery bypass grafting. Of the patients who died, 50% were in cardiogenic shock. Comparing coronary artery bypass grafting after failed angioplasty with elective coronary artery bypass grafting, the average number of grafts is 1.9 versus 2.6; with use of the internal thoracic artery, 9% versus 49%; with units of packed cells administered,

5.2% versus 3.3%; with incidence of acute myocardial infarction, 28% versus 9%; with bleeding, 28% versus 13%; with pericardial tamponade, 10.5% versus 1.5%; and with cardiac arrest, 6% versus 0%. The probability of angina 5 years following coronary artery bypass grafting after failed angioplasty is 21% versus 56% for angioplasty alone.

Reasonable indications for coronary balloon angioplasty include patients who refuse surgery; symptomatically disabled patients with widespread malignant or infectious disease processes; arteriosclerotic lesions that are concentric, noncalcified, away from branch points, and not in the most proximal portions of major coronary arteries; arteriosclerotic narrowing of a coronary artery responsible for disabling symptoms but supplying a functionally insignificant segment of myocardium; acute occlusion of a major coronary artery that has not responded to thrombolytic therapy; anastomotic narrowing of a coronary artery bypass graft; and severely compromised ventricular dysfunction that precludes surgical intervention.

The present case represented a high-risk angioplasty because of the proximal position of the lesion in the left anterior descending coronary artery. As illustrated by this case, the acute risks of dilating such a lesion include local dissection, retrodissection into the left main coronary artery, and propagation of a clot into the circumflex coronary artery. Because of the development of an acute left main equivalent lesion, the 80% lesion in the posterior descending was never addressed, creating a situation of incomplete revascularization. Although the patient remained marginally compensated with a bailout catheter, his myocardial reserve was now defined by significant lesions in all three major coronary vessels. Because of the acuity of the situation, this patient was denied the use of the internal thoracic artery as a graft for the left anterior descending coronary artery owing to the surgical team's reluctance to spend the extra time separating this vessel from the chest wall, despite the fact that this can be facilitated by using carbodissection of the pedicle; furthermore, the patient required three grafts instead of the two he would have required had he been operated electively.

Because procedural morbidity and mortality are a direct function of correct *de*cisions, not *in-*

cisions, whether or not a patient should undergo balloon angioplasty or coronary artery bypass grafting must be based on close collaboration between the cardiologist and the cardiac surgeon. The cardiologist must accept the reality that a patient who is a suitable candidate for surgery before angioplasty may not be a candidate for surgery after a failed angioplasty. The cardiac surgeon must insist upon an active role in this decision-making process, as he should decide the appropriateness of his involvement in any surgical procedure.

Having said this, it must be recognized that coronary artery bypass grafting is not a perfect procedure, either. Like angioplasty, it is palliative. Acute or chronic graft closure may occur (50% of vein grafts after 10 years, and 10% of internal thoracic artery grafts after 10 years). There are small but real risks of bleeding, stroke, infection, myocardial infarction, and insult to other organs, especially in patients over 80 years of age. For these reasons, many patients are advised to undergo coronary bal-loon angioplasty first, saving the coronary artery bypass procedure as a last resort. The major consideration in choosing any procedure must weigh the potential risks as opposed to the benefits; the issue is never, "I can do this," but must always be, "Should I do this?"

REFERENCES

1. Lee ME: How do you spell relief: PTCA or CABG? (letter). J Thorac Cardiovasc Surg 1989:97:935–936.
2. Connor AR, Vlietstra RE, Schaff HV, Ilstrup DM, Orszulak TA: Early and late results of coronary artery bypass after failed angioplasty: actuarial analysis of late cardiac events and comparison with initially successful angioplasty. J Thorac Cardiovasc Surg 1988:96:191–197.
3. Parsonnet V, Fisch D, Gielchinsky I, et al.: Emergency operation after failed angioplasty. J Thorac Cardiovasc Surg 1988:96:198–203.
4. Lee ME: Carbodissection of the internal thoracic artery pedicle. Ann Thorac Surg 1988: 46:470–471.

13

___

A 63-year-old patient with a strong family history of coronary artery disease presents with a one-year history of exertional angina. Cardiac catheterization reveals inferobasal akinesis, an 80% left main lesion, a 95% diagonal lesion, and total obstruction of the right coronary artery.

At surgery, you find a surprisingly large transmural infarction involving most of the posterior and inferior walls of the right and left ventricles. You graft the left internal thoracic artery to the left anterior descending and construct vein grafts to the diagonal, circumflex, and posterior descending coronary arteries. You separate the patient from cardiopulmonary bypass easily and transfer him to the cardiac surgical intensive care unit in satisfactory condition. You extubate the patient and remove the mediastinal drains and monitoring lines on the afternoon of the first postoperative day.

Later that evening, the patient spikes to 101.6° You obtain blood, sputum, and urine cultures. During this time, you notice a low systemic vascular resistance with a labile blood pressure, as well as oliguria and a rising serum creatine, for which you start a dopamine drip. By the morning of the second postoperative day, the patient requires reintubation for acute respiratory failure. Because of left lower lobe atelectasis, you perform a broncho-scopy to rule out a mucus plug. During the bronchoscopy, after a cough, you notice a small amount of serosanguineous fluid in the lower third of a totally benign appearing sternotomy incision. It is less than 48 hours after a completely uneventful operation and this patient now challenges you with his imminent self-destruction, making a cruel mockery of your best efforts. What should you do now?

SOLUTION

You obtain a gram stain of the sternal drainage and are shocked to find it reveals numerous gram-negative bacteria. Simultaneously, you learn that the blood cultures from the previous evening have grown out a gram-negative rod as well. The patient's white blood cell count has risen from 8900 on the first postoperative evening to 14,200. You start antibiotics and return the patient to the operating room without delay.

At surgery, you identify purulent material in the mediastinum and an acute fibrinous peel over the heart, as well as a 500 cc purulent effusion in the left pleural space. You irrigate the mediastinum, pericardium, and pleural space with 6 L of saline containing 5 cc/L of povidone-iodine (Betadine); place a chest tube in the pleural space; and place catheters for irrigation and drainage in the anterior mediastinum and posterior pericardium. You approximate the sternum with stainless steel wires and close the linea alba and pectoralis fascia with absorbable sutures. You pack the subcutaneous tissue with iodoform gauze and cover the incision with Betadine-impregnated plastic sheeting.

In the intensive care unit, you begin mediastinal irrigation with normal saline at 100 to 150 cc/hour and institute total parenteral nutrition. You administer industrial doses of organism-specific antibiotics. Despite this treatment, you identify a sternal dehiscence and return the patient to the operating room 8 days following his initial debridement for rotation of a pectoralis major muscle flap based on a thoracoacromial pedicle. The patient has a protracted course, but leaves the hospital and remains well, infection-free, a year and a half later.

DISCUSSION

The incidence of postoperative mediastinitis is 1% to 3% and is associated with a mortality rate of 25% with irrigation techniques alone. Although the etiology in this case was never identified, the rapid, almost ferocious, onset in this relatively young, healthy patient was consistent with a virtual inoculation at the time of surgery or in the intensive care unit. Contamination of the monitoring lines and injection ports, the injectate used to measure thermodilution cardiac outputs, the anesthesia cir-

cuit, the perfusion lines, or the surgical instruments were all possible sources.

Other causes that may predispose to such a complication include advanced age, poor nutritional status, diabetes mellitus, preexistent but subclinical infections, impaired immunocompetence, prolonged duration of surgery, low cardiac output, emergency reoperation for bleeding, use of both internal thoracic arteries for bypass conduits, and breaks in surgical technique. This patient's survival was a direct function of his otherwise excellent condition, the rapidity of the diagnosis and aggressive treatment, and support with parenteral nutrition from the beginning of his illness.

In the early days of cardiac surgery, the treatment of mediastinitis consisted of debridement, open drainage and packing, with slow granulation of the open wound over a period of weeks or months. More recently, debridement, sternal rewiring, and mediastinal irrigation with low concentration Betadine or antibiotic solutions has been successful but still carries a mortality rate of more than 20%. If this approach fails (as evidenced by recurrent culture-positive drainage and sternal dehiscence), rotation of pectoralis major or rectus abdominus muscle flaps, or omental transposition, after further debridement of devitalized soft tissue, cartilage, and bone, offer large volumes of viable tissue to fill dead space and restore stability to the chest wall. These techniques have reduced the mortality of postoperative mediastinitis to 5%.

REFERENCES

1. Shumaker HB, Mandelbaum I: Continuous antibiotic irrigation in the treatment of infection. Arch Surg 1963:86:384–387.
2. Bryant LR, Spencer FC, Trinkle JK: Treatment of median sternotomy infection by mediastinal irrigation with an antibiotic solution. Ann Surg 1969:169:914–920.
3. Scully HE, Leclerc Y, Martin RD, et al.: Comparison between antibiotic irrigation and mobilization of pectoral muscle flaps in treatment of deep sternal infections. J Thorac Cardiovasc Surg 1985:90:523–531.
4. Jurkiewicz MJ, Rand RP: The omentum in sternal wound reconstruction. Cardiac Surg 1988:2:475–484.

14

A 56-year-old patient with a history of angina pectoris and inter-mittent congestive heart failure for many years enters the hospital with pulmonary edema. Shortly after receiving an angiotensin-converting enzyme inhibitor to optimize afterload, the patient becomes hypotensive and develops angina pectoris with precordial ST segment elevation. In the cardiac catheterization laboratory, an intra-aortic balloon is inserted prior to angio-graphy. The left ventricular ejection fraction is 11% with contrac-tility observed only in the posterior wall, high septum, and base. A pedunculated, mobile clot is identified in the left ventricular apex. There is a 60% left main lesion, subtotal obstruction of the left anterior descending, which contains a mobile clot, subtotal obstruction of the obtuse circumflex marginal branches, and a congenitally small right coronary artery. You have been asked to evaluate the patient for surgery. An ejection fraction of 11%? They must be kidding!

SOLUTION

You decide that the basic issue is to determine whether or not the ventricular dysfunction is the result of scar or ischemia. You request a radionuclide wall motion study, which confirms the left ventricular ejection fraction of 11% and also reveals a right ventricular ejection fraction of 22%. Of considerable interest is a thallium study that demonstrates viable myocardium in all segments except the infero-apex, with normal wall thickness in both ventricles. Improvement in the cardiac index to 2.5 L/min/m^2 on a dobutamine drip in the absence of tachycardia, and recurrent chest pain with the discontinuation of nitroglycerine, suggest the presence of stunned myocardium as well as its capability for recruitment to enhance the patient's hemodynamics. The patient is certainly a candidate for revascularization. Your cardiologists decline to perform percutaneous transluminal coronary angioplasty because of the left main lesion, the complicated lesion in the left anterior descending, and the need for dilation of at least four vessels.

At surgery, with the appropriate caveats of high risk clearly understood by the patient and his family, you initially open the left ventricle and remove the apical clots to prevent their embolization during subsequent manipulation of the heart. You construct grafts to the left anterior descending, diagonal, and two circumflex branches. Separation from cardiopulmonary bypass is uneventful, and you are gratified to observe that the overall size of the heart is smaller with markedly improved contractility.

DISCUSSION

The key to appropriate decision making in this case rested upon the determination by clinical and laboratory parameters that this patient's cardiac dysfunction was largely ischemic. The literature documents that akinetic myocardial segments found to be viable with thallium scanning, and more recently with positron emission tomographic techniques, will demonstrate improved contractility after revascularization. That phenomenon was demonstrated in this case during surgery, admittedly with the patient under general anesthesia and with continuous monitoring of preload and afterload.

There is evidence that the more severe the left ventricular dysfunction, the greater the benefit of coronary bypass grafting, providing, of course, that reversible ischemia, and not diffuse scar, underlies much of the dysfunction, but early survival of these patients is lower than that of those with mildly depressed left ventricular function, especially if ventricular contractility does not improve quickly or completely enough to support the circulation. Pharmacologic and mechanical means of circulatory support, such as intra-aortic balloon counterpulsation or ventricular assist devices, may be necessary in such instances. According to the Coronary Artery Surgery Study, the 5-year surgical survival of patients with severe left ventricular dysfunction, three-vessel disease, and severe angina, is 69%, versus 32% for medically treated patients.

This patient could have been placed on a waiting list for cardiac transplantation based on his age and the absence of diabetes mellitus, infection, significant peripheral vascular disease, significant noncardiac illness, or pulmonary hypertension. This was not done because of the overwhelming evidence for reversible ventricular dysfunction. Furthermore, a recent study comparing coronary artery bypass grafting in transplant-eligible patients (group 1) versus transplant-ineligible patients (group 2), with a mean left ventricular ejection fraction of <30% in both groups, revealed no hospital deaths and a 3-year survival of 97% in group 1 and a 10% operative mortality and a 53% 3-year survival (p <.005) in group 2. The authors suggest that the results of cardiac transplantation must be compared to coronary artery bypass grafting in patients considered transplant eligible.

REFERENCES

1. Kirklin JW, et al.: Guidelines and indications for coronary artery bypass graft surgery: a report of the American College of Cardiology/American Heart Association task force on assessment of diagnostic and therapeutic cardiovascular procedures (subcommittee on coronary artery bypass graft surgery). J Am Coll Cardiol 1991:17:543–589.
2. Bateman T, Gray RJ, Czer LSC, Raymond MJ, Conklin CM, Maddahi J, Charuzi Y, Lee ME, Matloff JM, Berman D: The severely depressed left ventricle in ischemic heart disease: rest-redistribution Tl-201 imaging predicts improvement after revascularization (abstract). J Nucl Med 1986:27:933.

3. Geltman EM: Positron emission tomography. Cardio November 1987:77–84.
4. Califf RM, Harrell FE Jr, Lee KL, et al.: The evolution of medical and surgical therapy for coronary artery disease. A 15 year perspective. JAMA 1989:261:2077–2086.
5. Myers WO, Gersh BJ, Fisher LD, et al.: Medical versus early surgical therapy in patients with triple-vessel disease and mild angina pectoris: a CASS registry study of survival. Ann Thorac Surg 1987:44:471–486.
6. Stout MJ, Cheung EH, Letson B, Hatcher CR Jr, Guyton RA: Coronary bypass is superior to transplantation for patients with angina and poor LV function (abstract). Chest August 1990 supplement.

15

A 65-year-old patient undergoes reoperation for coronary artery disease. On the fifth postoperative day, the patient becomes febrile with an elevated white count, and purulent material (which subsequently grew out *Staphylococcus aureus*) drains from the sternotomy incision. Mediastinal exploration with debridement, sternal rewiring, and subsequent mediastinal irrigation with a dilute solution of povidone-iodine (Betadine) is carried out for 6 days, after which the mediastinal drains are removed. Twelve hours later, at 2:45 A.M., you receive a call from the intensive care unit nurse who frantically tells you the patient has incurred a massive hemorrhage from the lower part of the sternotomy incision, and that his blood pressure has fallen to 80 mm Hg. The patient has also sustained several seconds of asystole but stabilized with a brief period of closed chest massage and volume infusion. As you stumble into your car, you are tormented by a bittersweet conflict: (1) how great it will be to race down an empty freeway at 90 miles an hour! and (2) I think I'd rather be in bed!

SOLUTION

At surgery, you identify a few mediastinal clots. Removal of one of them results in brisk bleeding from the toe of the circumflex proximal anastomosis. Despite your apprehension that the tissues might be friable, your pledgeted mattress suture holds. You freshen up the edges of the incision and close it, insert the chest tubes, and pack the subcutaneous tissue with iodoform gauze.

Feeling elated with the results of your efforts, you both make it through the day, thinking that if it had been the aortic cannulation site, you and the patient might not have been so lucky. You retire early, expecting a good night's sleep but have a nightmare that the telephone is ringing and the intensive care unit nurse is telling you the patient has suddenly dumped a liter of blood from his chest tubes. As you ascend to a higher level of consciousness, you realize the telephone *is* ringing, it is 1:45 A.M., and the nurse on the line *is* pleading with you to wake up and get to the hospital right away. You are hard pressed to accept this two nights in a row and lapse into paranoid ideation, muttering, "Why is this patient doing this to me after all I've done for him?" as you lurch to the garage and start the car.

At surgery, you find another bleeding point, this time at the toe of the left anterior descending graft, and control it with a single suture. The repair from the previous night remains intact. The remainder of the patient's hospital course is uneventful and the patient remains well more than 5 years postoperatively.

DISCUSSION

The causes of postoperative mediastinitis have been partially reviewed elsewhere in this volume. They include, as well, prolonged operative time, prolonged postoperative respiratory insufficiency, obesity, and improper handling of tissues such as excessive use of the cautery or suture lines closed under tension with strangulating sutures. An additional factor in this patient was the administration of a short course of steroids in the initial postoperative period. Steroids had been given to prevent a recurrence of pericarditis, which was thought to have contributed to graft closure after this patient's first bypass operation several years previously.

Infections involving vascular suture lines can be acutely or chronically catastrophic. Infection of the aortic cannulation site in this patient would probably have been fatal, as would have been a complete dehiscence of a proximal anastomosis. More chronic manifestations of infection can present as an anastomotic false aneurysm or as endocarditis causing dehiscence of prosthetic valves, annular abscesses, or disturbances in the cardiac conduction system.

REFERENCES

1. Ottino G, De Paulis R, Pansini S, Rocca G, Tallone MV, Comoglio C, Costa P, Orzan F, Morea M: Major sternal wound infection after open heart surgery: a multivariate analysis of risk factors in 2579 consecutive operative procedures. Ann Thorac Surg 1987:44:173–179.
2. Demmy TL, Park SB, Liebler GA, Burkholder JA, Maher TD, Benckart DH, Magovern GJ Jr, Magovern GJ Sr: Recent experience with major sternal wound complications. Ann Thorac Surg 1990:49:458–462.
3. Spencer FC, Grossi EA: Mediastinitis after cardiac operations (key references). Ann Thorac Surg 1990:49:506–507.

16

_____

A 72-year-old patient presents with a 2-day history of chest pain. The electrocardiogram reveals an evolving anterior myocardial infarction, and there is biochemical evidence that the patient is on the downward slope of what must have been an earlier rise in his creatine phosphokinase level. On the day following admission, 3 days following the onset of chest pain, a harsh precordial murmur appears. Doppler echocardiography documents a ventricular septal defect with a left-to-right shunt. Cardiac catheterization confirms the presence of a ventricular septal defect with a Qp:Qs of 3:1. There is total obstruction of the left anterior descending coronary artery. The diagonal and a large circumflex coronary artery are normal, and a large right coronary artery has mild diffuse disease. The patient is reasonably stable on a dopamine drip with a heart rate in the 90s but is beginning to develop congestive heart failure. You have been asked to guide this patient's management.

SOLUTION

Despite the fact that the ventricular septal defect occurred about 3 days following the myocardial infarction and the involved tissues will be soft and necrotic, you elect to operate urgently before further heart and multisystem organ failure ensue. You feel encouraged because the patient has not, as yet, required intra-aortic balloon counterpulsation for circulatory support.

At surgery, you identify an acute anterolateral-apical infarction and palpate a thrill at the lower aspect of the right ventricular free wall. You open the left ventricle through the infarction to the left of the interventricular septum, identify the septal defect, and remove all necrotic septal tissue, unroofing the septum as you enter the right ventricle. Fortunately, the papillary muscle of the tricuspid valve appears not to be involved.

You next cut a circular patch of filamentous Dacron, fold it over on itself, and place it so as to straddle the interventricular septum, with the folded edge allowed to protrude through the ventriculotomy. You pass multiple pledgeted mattress sutures through both sides of the patch as it straddles the septum, the sutures passing through the septum as far from the debrided edge as possible. You then place Teflon felt strips along the edges of the biventriculotomy and pass sutures through the strips, the cut edges of the ventricles, and through the folded part of the patch, which protrudes through the incision. Once you terminate cardiopulmonary bypass, an intraoperative Doppler echocardiogram confirms complete repair of the defect.

DISCUSSION

Postinfarction ventricular septal defects account for 5% of all postinfarction deaths. With medical management alone, a postinfarction ventricular septal defect has a 2-month mortality of about 75% and a 1-year survival of 5% or less. They usually result from acute total occlusion of a large single vessel, most frequently the left anterior descending, in the presence of a small right coronary artery, which results in an antero-apical defect. Somewhat less frequently, a large right coronary artery in the presence of a small left anterior descending becomes occluded, resulting in a posterior septal-apical defect. The latter lesion has a higher operative mortality because of the higher associated incidence of right ventricular dysfunction, and the possible requirement for additional intervention that results from ischemia or infarction of the papillary muscles of the mitral valve.

The onset of a postinfarction ventricular septal defect is usually 3 to 5 days after the initial event and is associated with acute hemodynamic decompensation that frequently requires endotracheal intubation because of pulmonary edema, as well as circulatory support with inotropes and intra-aortic balloon counterpulsation. The differential diagnosis between acute ventricular septal defect and a ruptured papillary muscle of the mitral valve can be determined by insertion of a Swan-Ganz pulmonary artery catheter with simultaneous measurement of the right atrial, pulmonary arterial, and systemic arterial oxygen saturations. A stepup in oxygen saturation in the right ventricle or the pulmonary artery confirms the diagnosis of a ventricular septal defect. The diagnosis may be made more rapidly and noninvasively with Doppler echocardiography. Cardiac catheterization to determine the coronary anatomy need be performed only if the condition of the patient is stable.

Cooley et al. reported the first surgical repair of a postinfarction ventricular septal defect, and Kitamura et al. reported a 32% survival after one year. Because of high early operative mortality rates, initial efforts at repair were delayed as long as possible to allow infarcted tissue to develop scar capable of holding sutures, but only patients with smaller, restrictive defects could survive this delay in treatment. As newer techniques of patching ventricular septal defects in conjunction with patch reconstruction of the posterior and inferior ventricular walls to reduce tension on the suture lines evolved, repairs were attempted earlier in the course of the disease. Postinfarction ventricular septal defect is now regarded as an indication for acute surgical intervention. Using the method described in the present case, a tension-free repair of any antero-apical septal defect can be performed at any postinfarction time interval with a 30 day mortality of less than 20%. The repair of ventricular septal defects associated with posteroinferior infarcts has a significantly higher operative mortality (60%) especially if cardiogenic shock and transventricular mitral valve repair or replacement are required as additional procedures.

REFERENCES

1. Fox AC, Glassman E, Ison OW: Surgically remediable complications of myocardial infarction. Prog Cardiovasc Dis 1979:21:461–484.
2. Cooley DA, Belmonte BA, Zeis LB, Schnur S: Surgical repair of ruptured interventricular septum following acute myocardial infarction. Surgery 1957:41:930–937.
3. Kitamura S, Mendez A, Kay JH: Ventricular septal defect following myocardial infarction. J Thorac Cardiovasc Surg 1971:61:186–199.
4. Miyamoto A, Lee ME, Kass RM, et al.: Post-myocardial infarction ventricular septal defect. J Thorac Cardiovasc Surg 1983:86:41–46.
5. Daggett WM, Guyton RA, Mundth ED, et al.: Surgery for postmyocardial infarct ventricular septal defect. Ann Surg 1977:186:260–271.
6. Radford MJ, Johnson RA, Daggett WM, et al.: Ventricular septal rupture: a review of clinical and physiologic features and an analysis of survival. Circulation 1981:64:545–553.
7. Moore CA, Nygaard TW, Kaiser DL, et al.: Post infarction ventricular septal rupture: the importance of location and right ventricular function in determining survival. Circulation 1986:74:45–55.
8. Jones MT, Schofield PM, Dark JF, et al.: Surgical repair of acquired ventricular septal defect. J Thorac Cardiovasc Surg 1987:93:680–686.
9. Gray RJ, Sethna DH, Matloff JM: The role of cardiac surgery in acute myocardial infarction I. with mechanical defects. Am Heart J 1983: 106:723–728.

17

___

An obese 83-year-old patient has been admitted with acute pulmonary edema. Doppler echocardiography reveals 4⁺ mitral insufficiency, excellent left ventricular contractility, and normal coronary arteries, but the patient refuses surgical intervention. A short time after her catheterization, the patient requires transfer to the intensive care unit because of the sudden onset of hypotension, tachypnea, and tachycardia, thought to have resulted from a ruptured chorda tendina. Physical examination reveals persistence of the mitral insufficiency murmur with a few bibasilar rales. You recommend an emergency operation.

At surgery, the heart rate is 110, the right atrial pressure is 29 mm Hg, and the cardiac index is 1.3 L/min/m². The patient sustains another episode of profound hypotension shortly after endotracheal intubation. You perform rapid sternotomy and cannulate with a 24 Fr. aortic perfusion cannula and a 51–36 double-caged venous drainage cannula.

The great vessels are normal, the right atrium somewhat dilated, and the ventricles of normal size and contractility with no evidence of transmural infarction. Almost immediately after you begin cardiopulmonary bypass, your perfusionist informs you of a rapidly falling blood level in the oxygenator and that he has reached the point where he is no longer able to maintain adequate perfusion. You feel that bone-chilling numbness that rises from your feet and courses through your body right to the fingertips when you sense that something is terribly wrong and everyone is watching.

SOLUTION

You notice that the right side of the heart has become dramatically dilated and is not being decompressed by the venous cannula. You quickly ascertain there are no kinks in the venous line, no clamps on the line, and the tip of the venous cannula to be in the proper position, with its tip in the inferior vena cava. As you palpate the vena cava, however, you sense it has a spongy, soft feel, and decide that, no matter what is going on, you are going to replace the two-stage cannula with separate superior and inferior vena cava cannulas. You place a pledgeted purse-string suture at the junction of the superior vena cava with the right atrium, place two single-stage venous drainage cannulas onto a Y connector, and interrupt cardiopulmonary bypass. You clamp the two-stage venous cannula and, with a clamp on the new inferior vena cava cannula, insert the other cannula into the superior vena cava and restore venous return to the oxygenator. As you remove the two-stage cannula, you are amazed to see that it is followed by four separate organized thrombi, each 10 cm long and 1 cm in diameter. You quickly insert the new inferior vena cava cannula and restore full flow with marked decompression of the right side of the heart.

DISCUSSION

Impaired right-sided decompression in this case resulted from occlusion of a two-stage venous drainage cannula by multiple emboli from the pelvic veins and deep venous system of the lower extremities. It is likely that the patient's episodes of hypotension that precipitated both her arrival in the operating room and the necessity for rapid entry into the chest shortly after intubation resulted from recurrent pulmonary emboli. The fact that only mild bibasilar rales could be heard just prior to transfer to the operating room was more consistent with this diagnosis than with an exacerbation of mitral insufficiency, which should have been associated with florid pulmonary edema, despite the aggressiveness of any prior diuresis. The mitral valve itself revealed only myxomatous degeneration.

Other causes of impaired venous return include malpositioning of a two-stage cannula such that its tip is in the right ventricle instead of the inferior vena cava, or perforation of the inferior vena cava by the tip of the cannula with the cannula itself obstructing flow from the vena cava. Even with two separate venous cannulas, impaired venous return can result from snaring of the superior and/or inferior vena cava with tapes placed beyond the tips of the cannulas, effectively ligating the venae cavae. It can also result from failure to drain blood from a left superior vena cava draining into the coronary sinus or placement of the cannulas too far into the cavae so as to obstruct venous return from the azygous vein or the hepatic veins. Common to both methods of cannulation, impaired venus drainage may result from kinks in the venous line; a clamp left on the venous line; an air lock that impedes gravity drainage into the oxygenator with air entry into the line from around an atrial purse-string suture or from an unrecognized tear, usually at the junction of the innominate vein with the superior vena cava; or an acute intraoperative aortic dissection.

REFERENCES

1. Dalen JE, Alpert JS: Pulmonary embolism, in Hurst JW, Logue RB, Schlant RC, Sonnenblick EH, Wallace AG, Wenger NK, eds., *The Heart*, sixth edition. New York: McGraw-Hill Book Company, 1986, pages 1105–1119.
2. Kurusz M, Wheeldon DR: Risk containment during cardiopulmonary bypass. Seminars in Thorac and Cardiovasc Surg 1990:2:400–409.

18

A 66-year-old patient who had undergone coronary artery bypass grafting 12 years previously, enters the hospital for the evaluation and treatment of ventricular arrhythmias. One year prior to admission, the patient had been started on quinidine because of premature ventricular contractions. He was subsequently admitted because of syncope. An electrophysiology study revealed sick sinus syndrome with no inducible ventricular tachycardia, and a bipolar SSI pacemaker was implanted. Three months prior to the present admission, the patient experienced polymorphic ventricular tachycardia refractory to multiple antiarrhythmic agents and was finally placed on amiodarone. While controlling the arrhythmia, this treatment caused severe pulmonary insufficiency that necessitated cessation of the amiodarone and endotracheal intubation for a 3-week period. During this time, the pO_2 was in the 40s and the patient required pharmacologic circulatory support. Since extubation, the patient has had an intermittent, nonproductive dry cough.

Although the patient has not had any recent clinical episodes of ventricular tachycardia, probably because of high residual amiodarone tissue levels, another electrophysiology study demonstrates inducible ventricular tachycardia, which degenerates into ventricular fibrillation. Cardiac catheterization reveals antero-apical and apical-inferior akinesis. There is total obstruction of the left anterior descending and right coronary arteries with a relatively normal circumflex. Grafts to the left anterior descending and right coronary arteries are patent. You are consulted to implant an automatic implantable cardioverter- defibrillator (AICD).

On physical examination, you are startled to find diffuse dry rales throughout both lung fields. A chest roentgenogram reveals a prominent bilateral reticular pattern consistent with interstitial fibrosis. Pulmonary function studies reveal a diffusion capacity of 43%, with room air arterial blood gases showing a pH of 7.38, pCO_2 of 41, and a pO_2 of 72. What is your recommendation?

SOLUTION

Because of the high operative mortality rate of any surgical procedure that requires general anesthesia in patients with residual amiodarone-induced pulmonary dysfunction, you urge your electrophysiologist to consider other modalities of treatment: (1) trials of other antiarrhythmic drugs in an attempt to provide time for further resolution of the pulmonary dysfunction; (2) transfer of the patient to a center investigating AICD systems employing transvenous rate sensing leads and transvenous and subcutaneous defibrillating leads, all of which can be implanted using local anesthetics without a thoracotomy; (3) an attempt at radio frequency catheter ablation of the arrythmogenic focus in the left ventricle, recognizing that the success of such a procedure is currently only between 30% and 50% and has risks that include perforation of the ventricle and cerebrovascular accident. The next morning, after what you had considered to be a thoughtful approach, you discover that the patient has been transferred to another institution for implantation of a conventional AICD through a left thoracotomy incision under general anesthesia.

The patient receives pretreatment with corticosteroids. Anesthesia includes induction by sufentanil and thiopental (Pentothal), with maintenance by isoflurane (Forane), and a 5 to 6 L flow of oxygen, sufficient to maintain an oxygen saturation ranging between 94% and 100%. The patient is extubated promptly following the procedure, with analgesia provided by epidural duramorph. Within 48 hours, the patient becomes dyspneic, hypoxemic, and requires endotracheal intubation at a time when the arterial blood gases reveal a pH of 7.20, a pCO_2 of 50, and a pO_2 of 20. The intubation is difficult and is complicated by a cardiac arrest from which the patient is resuscitated but remains comatose from anoxic encephalopathy until his demise 14 days later.

DISCUSSION

Amiodarone is a potent antiarrhythmic drug that slows repolarization and increases the fibrillatory threshold in myocardial cells. It is slowly absorbed, is protein bound, and has an elimination half-life estimated to be between 10 and 50 days. Pulmonary abnormalities appear to be dose and/or duration related, especially in patients who receive maintenance doses of greater than 400 mg daily over a period of 14 months, and are more common in patients with preexistent pulmonary dysfunction. Patients may present with interstitial or alveolar infiltrates, which may progress with startling rapidity to a respiratory distress syndrome characterized by pulmonary edema and hemorrhage, hyaline membrane formation, and superimposed infections. Because of its long half-life, significant amounts of amiodarone and its metabolite, desethylamiodarone, may persist in pulmonary tissue long after symptomatic and radiographic improvement has occurred. As illustrated by this case, it is typical for such patients to be extubated following an uneventful general anesthetic, only to experience the rapid progression of respiratory insufficiency.

Many factors, in addition to preexistent pulmonary dysfunction, have been suspected to increase the risk of deterioration of pulmonary function in patients who have received amiodarone. These include inspired oxygen, especially in concentrations greater than 60%; anesthetic agents; and cardiopulmonary bypass. Because of the extremely high operative mortality rate, patients with a history of amiodarone ingestion with known spirometric or diffusion abnormalities of pulmonary function should not be subjected to any procedure that requires general anesthesia.

The treatment of amiodarone pulmonary toxicity is nonspecific and includes cessation of the drug, administration of corticosteroids, diuresis, and mechanical ventilatory support with the lowest concentration possible of inspired O_2 to reduce the added insult of oxygen toxicity. Whether the employment of venovenous extracorporeal membrane oxygenation (ECMO) has a role in supporting these patients has not been demonstrated.

This case is another illustration of the fact that surgical morbidity and mortality rates are a direct function of correct *de*cisionmaking, not correct *in*cision making.

REFERENCES

1. McGovern B, Garon H, Ruskin JM: Serious adverse effects of amiodarone. Clin Cardiol 1984:7:131–137.

2. Schecter CJ, O'Neill G, Schweppe HI Jr, et al.: Asymptomatic cavitary pneumonitis due to amiodarone pulmonary toxicity. Texas Heart Inst J 1985:12:371–375.

3. Nalos PC, Kass RM, Gang ES, et al.: Life-threatening postoperative pulmonary complications in patients with previous amiodarone pulmonary toxicity undergoing cardiothoracic operations. J Thorac Cardiovasc Surg 1987:93:904–912.

4. Lee ME: Pulmonary Care, in Gray RJ, Matloff JM, eds. *Medical Management of the Cardiac Surgical Patient*, Baltimore: Williams and Wilkins, 1990, pages 164–173.

19

A 66-year-old patient enters the hospital with crescendo angina. Nine years previously he underwent coronary artery bypass grafting, which had been complicated by an angiographically proven pulmonary embolus. Cardiac catheterization reveals satisfactory left ventricular function, subtotal obstruction of the left anterior descending and right coronary arteries, total occlusion of the left anterior descending and diagonal grafts, an 80% narrowing in the circumflex graft, and a 95% lesion in the right coronary graft.

Your preoperative evaluation reveals that both greater saphenous veins had previously been used. A duplex scan shows the lesser saphenous veins to be small. You begin the operation by harvesting cephalic veins from both arms, reprep and redrape, and enter the chest. You free up the aorta and right atrium, take down the left internal thoracic artery, cannulate, and then begin to dissect out the remainder of the heart from the adhesions. An ominous spurt of red blood appears and you just *know* you've transsected the left anterior descending. You institute cardiopulmonary bypass at once, confident of being able to protect the myocardium with your antegrade and retrograde cardioplegia delivery systems.

You construct cephalic vein grafts to the diagonal, two circumflexes, and the right posterior descending, and then a sequential left anterior descending–left anterior descending internal thoracic artery graft proximal and distal to the point of transsection of the left anterior descending coronary artery. After rewarming, you are pleased to be able to separate the patient from cardiopulmonary bypass easily. It has been a trying case, and you just want to sit down and put your feet up.

You give the protamine, decannulate, secure hemostasis, implant the pacing wires, and place the mediastinal drains. As you begin to tie the sternal wires, thankful the case has come to a successful conclusion, you notice the patient has become profoundly bradycardic, with a heart rate of 35, and hypotensive as well. What now?

SOLUTION

As you rapidly untie the sternal wires, you can't help but wonder whether the patient could have had another pulmonary embolus. With the sternal retractor in place, you immediately notice three things: the heart is dilated, cyanotic, and diffusely hypocontractile; the blood in the vein grafts is black; the lungs are not moving. You alert the anesthesiologist as you begin to massage the heart. You keep repeating that the patient is not being ventilated. The blood is black, the lungs are not moving, he is not being ventilated!

Your impassioned repetition of these words begin to have an effect. The anesthesiologist tries bagging the patient by hand, but senses resistance to air entry. He begins troubleshooting the system by looking under the drapes and immediately spots the kink in the endotracheal tube which had fallen off its support. Once corrected, ventilation becomes easy again, the lungs begin to move, the grafts pink up, and contractility improves. The remainder of the patient's course is uneventful.

DISCUSSION

The key to the successful resolution of this problem was rapid reentry into the chest. This enabled diagnostic and therapeutic measures to proceed at once. One must avoid the temptation to focus attention only on the heart as a primary cause of the difficulty but, rather, run through a cardiopulmonary checklist, especially since bypass had been terminated easily. The diffuse hypocontractility and black blood in the bypass grafts could only have resulted from impaired ventilation because exploration of the chest revealed neither lung to be moving. Despite the fact that the initial intubation was successful, as documented by clear visualization of the vocal cords, good bilateral motion of the chest, good bilateral breath sounds, and normal end-tidal CO_2 determinations, it is

essential that the anesthesiologist quickly overcome any initial reaction of disbelief and denial and identify the source of the problem without delay.

Other causes of sudden hypoventilation include dislodgement of the endotracheal tube proximal to the vocal cords with the tip buried in, or perforating, the pyriform sinus; displacement of the tube into an endobronchial position, causing profound intrapulmonary shunting in the nonventilated lung; deflation of the endotracheal tube cuff, causing a massive air leak; detachment of the endotracheal tube from the ventilator; ball-valve plugging of the endotracheal tube with a mucus plug, clot, or foreign body; and tension pneumothorax. Special attention must be given to the endotracheal tube when turning the head from side to side during cardiopulmonary bypass, when turning the patient to a different position, and when transferring the patient from the operating room table to a bed for the move to the intensive care unit.

Other considerations in this patient included recurrent, acute pulmonary embolus; a myocardial infarction perhaps secondary to a kinked vein graft, for which there was neither hemodynamic nor electrocardiographic evidence; and, certainly, the possibility of a protamine reaction especially in a patient with prior exposure to protamine.

This case provides ample illustration of the indispensability of constant vigilance and the undisputed importance of constantly working under the assumption that if something can go wrong, it will, and at the most inauspicious or unguarded moment.

REFERENCES

1. Hensley FA Jr, Larach DR, Martin DE: Intraoperative anesthetic complications and their management, in Waldhausen JA, Orringer MB, eds. *Complications in Cardiothoracic Surgery*, St. Louis, MO: Mosby Year Book, 1991, pages 3–19.

20

A 66-year-old patient enters the hospital with congestive heart failure secondary to an acute anterolateral myocardial infarction. At cardiac catheterization, the left ventricular end-diastolic pressure is 25 mm Hg. There is akinesis of the anterolateral and apical segments of the left ventricle, total obstruction of the left anterior descending coronary artery beyond a large septal perforator, total obstruction of the circumflex coronary artery, an ulcerated plaque in the right coronary artery proximal to the right ventricular marginal branch, and total obstruction of the distal right coronary artery with left-to-right collateralization of the distal right coronary branches from the first diagonal.

At surgery, a left radial arterial line is inserted and a Swan-Ganz pulmonary artery catheter advanced to the wedge position through the right internal jugular vein. Upon opening the pericardium, you observe anterolateral and apical akinesis but no evidence of transmural myocardial infarction. You graft the left anterior descending with the left internal thoracic artery, graft the right ventricular marginal with the right internal thoracic artery, and use vein grafts for the circumflex marginal, right posterior descending, and right posterolateral coronary arteries. After rewarming, de-airing, and termination of cardiopulmonary bypass, the cardiac output remains low in the presence of high filling pressures. Despite institution of pharmacologic circulatory support, hypocontractility of not only the anterolateral segments of the left ventricle but also of the right ventricular free wall persists, and you decide to employ intra-aortic balloon counterpulsation.

You place the balloon on the chest wall and measure off a length extending from the femoral insertion site to 2 cm below the supra sternal notch. This ensures that the balloon will not impinge upon the orifice of the left subclavian artery and possibly interfere with measurement of the radial artery pressure. Using the percutaneous technique, you advance a 9.5 Fr. intra-aortic balloon through a long sheath into the descending thoracic aorta. You withdraw the sheath far enough to clear the balloon, inflate the balloon with a syringe to ensure that it has unfurled, and connect it to the console. To your surprise, despite apparently normal function of the console, you do not see diastolic augmentation in the arterial pressure trace. You must solve this problem before the patient deteriorates any further.

SOLUTION

You ask your balloon technician to trouble-shoot the console. The console has been set to trigger from the electrocardiogram and is receiving a tracing of appropriate quality and amplitude. The helium tanks are full and the valves open, with no evidence of volume loss. The balloon has been set to inflate at a 1:1 ratio with the maximum volume of helium delivered to the balloon with each cycle. There are no kinks in the lines. As the patient continues to deteriorate, you palpate the ascending aorta once again and confirm the absence of diastolic augmentation in the presence of apparently normal console function.

In mounting frustration, you happen to notice the reflection of the operating room lights on the surface of the right atrium and that the atrium appears to have extra activity not reflected in the electrocardiogram. In disbelief, you put your hand on the atrium and palpate a throbbing mass! Knowing now that the balloon had entered the femoral vein and found its way to the right atrium, it is a simple matter to enter the femoral artery and redirect the balloon to its proper position in the proximal descending thoracic aorta whereupon you observe perfect augmentation. The patient makes an uneventful recovery.

DISCUSSION

It is occasionally difficult to be certain whether the femoral artery or vein has been entered when perioperative balloon pumping must be instituted in the presence of hypotension, depressed cardiac output, and hypoxemia. If the patient is on bypass, there will be no pulsation in the femoral artery and venous blood may appear quite red. Patients considered to be likely candidates for balloon counterpulsation should have the initial monitoring of their systemic blood pressure through a femoral arterial line rather than a radial artery line in order to establish femoral arterial access under controlled circumstances.

REFERENCES

1. Richenbacher WE, Pierce WS: Management of complications of intraaortic balloon counterpulsation in Waldhausen JA, Orringer MB, eds.; *Complications in Cardiothoracic Surgery*, St Louis, MO: Mosby Year Book, 1991, pages 97–102.
2. Summers D, Kaplitt M, Norris J, Rubin R, Nacht R, Arieff A, Lee ME, Wechsler B, Sawyer PN: Intra-aortic balloon pumping: hemodynamic and metabolic effects during cardiogenic shock in patients with triple-coronary artery obstructive disease. Arch Surg 1969:99:733–738.

21

A 40-year-old patient underwent resection of a fibrosarcoma of the left forearm. Two years later, he requires a right pneumonectomy for metastatic disease. Six days prior to the present admission the patient experiences inspiratory and expiratory dyspnea, especially worse when he lay on his back. On physical examination there is marked stridor. Roentgenographic examination of the airway reveals a large pedunculated mass attached to the anterior wall of the distal trachea. Flexible fiberoptic bronchoscopy is performed using topical anesthesia. This demonstrates a large mass that almost completely obstructs the left main-stem bronchus. During this evaluation, the patient becomes acutely dyspneic and cyanotic. Rapid endotracheal intubation is performed, which provides some degree of ventilation but with extremely high airway pressure. You are asked to consult on an emergency basis.

SOLUTION

You had actually been aware of this case prior to the time bronchoscopy was performed. You quickly expose the common femoral artery and vein, cannulate them, and place the patient on cardiopulmonary bypass. You achieve excellent oxygenation with flows between 2.5 and 3.0 L/min. Once this degree of stability has been achieved, laser ablation of the tumor proceeds uneventfully.

DISCUSSION

Management of the acute airway obstruction in this patient was facilitated by your preoperative awareness of a specific lesion and availability of the cardiac surgical team on a standby basis. With a ball-valve type of lesion obstructing ventilation to the only remaining lung, cardiopulmonary bypass was the only means of ventilating and resuscitating this patient.

Functional or anatomic airway obstruction may occur at any time in the perioperative period and at any anatomic level of the respiratory tract. Among the numerous etiologies are contact of the base of the tongue with the posterior oropharynx, laryngospasm, anatomic abnormalities of the upper airway, inflammatory or neoplastic lesions of the retropharynx or airway structures themselves, traumatic disruption of the airway, foreign bodies, chronic obstructive pulmonary disease, diffusion abnormalities of the lung, tension pneumothorax, flail chest, and restrictive chest wall disease.

It is critical to recall that even with assured placement of an endotracheal tube in the trachea, as documented by visualization of its passage through the vocal cords, that obstruction of the tube may occur by displacement, kinking, or obstruction by secretions. Recently, a manufacturing defect in a double-lumen endotracheal tube was described in which a semicircular protrusion of plastic significantly obstructed one of the lumens. It was discovered with a fiberoptic bronchoscope used to confirm the position of the tube, which was quickly changed.

The treatment of airway obstruction depends upon the cause. In general, muscle relaxants are not given unless ventilation by a mask is possible. Mask ventilation may be followed by attempts at intubation using a conventional laryngoscope, nasal intubation, flexible fiberoptic-assisted intubation, intubation over a guide wire passed proximally into the oropharynx through a Tuohy needle inserted through the cricothyroid membrane, tracheostomy, and less commonly employed techniques such as veno-venous extracorporeal membrane oxygenation, or cardiopulmonary bypass using rapid percutaneous cannulation techniques.

REFERENCES

1. Hensley FA Jr, Larach DR, Martin DE: Intraoperative anesthetic complications and their management, in Waldhausen JA, Orringer MB, eds., *Complications in Cardiothoracic Surgery*, St. Louis, MO: Mosby Year Book, 1991 pages 3–19.
2. Barash PG, Cullen BF, Stoelting RK, eds., *Clinical Anesthesia*, Philadelphia: J.B.Lippincott Company, 1989.
3. Campbell C, Viswanathan S, Riopelle JM, Naraghi M: Manufacturing defect in a double-lumen tube. Anesthesia and Analgesia 1991:73:825-826
4. Zwischenberger JB, Bartlett RH: Extracorporeal circulation for respiratory or cardiac failure. Seminars in Thorac and Cardiovasc Surg 1990:2:320–331.

Lagniappe

A 65-year-old patient with severe calcific aortic stenosis undergoes a smooth induction and endotracheal intubation in preparation for aortic valve replacement. Shortly after intubation, there is
high airway pressure associated with diminished chest wall ex-
cursions, distant breath sounds, and progressive cyanosis. There
is no question that the tube is in the trachea and there are no perceived abnormalities of the anesthesia circuit. You and your anesthesiologist quickly concur that the tube must be pulled and stare
in disbelief at the tooth, one of the patient's upper incisors,
caught in the Murphy side hole of the endotracheal tube, virtually obstructing the airway! After a brief period of ventilation by
mask, reintubation is performed and you complete the remainder of the procedure uneventfully.

22

A 60-year-old patient with progressive angina is found to have triple vessel disease in need of coronary artery bypass grafting. In the operating room, the patient maintains normal hemodynamics during a smooth anesthetic induction, endotracheal intubation, prepping, draping, and sternotomy. You perform routine cannulations of the ascending aorta, insert a two-stage venous drainage cannula into the right atrium and the inferior vena cava, and a catheter into the ascending aorta to serve as an aortic root vent and as a conduit for the antegrade administration of cardioplegia. You begin cardiopulmonary bypass and prepare to put the finishing touches on the internal thoracic artery pedicle while waiting for core cooling and application of the aortic crossclamp. The anesthesiologist has just started playing the overture to "Swan Lake" and you are settling down for what should be a pleasant few hours when your perfusionist intrudes upon this idyll saying that he can't maintain a mean pressure over 30 mm Hg and that during these few horrifying seconds his oxygenator has filled and is quickly overflowing into the cardiotomy reservoir.

SOLUTION

Since the heart is empty, you know there cannot be a problem with impaired venous return. The ascending aorta appears normal, and you cannot palpate anything that feels like a dissected aorta through the posterior pericardium. As you turn around to look at the amazing sight in the oxygenator, the perfusionist spots the problem: You have neglected to clamp the recirculation shunt between the arterial and venous lines. You quickly grab a tubing clamp, apply it to the line, grateful to see the perfusion pressure rise and the level in the oxygenator fall as the curtain rises on act one of "Swan Lake." At this point, you feel like an unwelcomed guest at Siegfried's birthday party, though the remainder of your case proceeds as you had originally intended.

DISCUSSION

If one accepts the premise that human error is responsible for most complications relating to cardiopulmonary bypass rather than equipment malfunction, then it becomes apparent that consistently excellent results derive from rigid adherence to a single standard protocol for all open heart procedures performed at a single institution. This means that all members of the heart team function in concert, using similar approaches to monitoring, techniques of anesthesia, instrument trays, and perfusion set-up. It also means that patterns of interaction among anesthesiologist, surgeon, perfusionist, and nurses remain constant and predictable from case to case. The administration of anesthetic agents and vasoactive drugs during bypass must be shared between the anesthesiologist and the perfusionist. The anesthesiologist must know to lower the blood pressure before aortic cannulation and prepare to elevate it in anticipation of the bleed back. The perfusionist must lower the perfusion pressure in anticipation of aortic crossclamping and declamping. The scrub nurse should know enough of every procedure in order to anticipate the next step and thereby maintain the smooth rhythm created by the swift, silent passage of instruments from one hand to the other.

Each specialist within the team must follow a mental or written checklist to be sure nothing is forgotten or done out of sequence: the anesthesiologist and the preoperative check of his machine and preparation of drugs, the perfusionist and his setting up of the pump-oxygenator. If heparin is given by the anesthesiologist, the surgeon should request it at the appropriate time. If the surgeon forgets to ask for it, the anesthesiologist must remind the surgeon and then acknowledge it has been given. The perfusionist must not allow bypass to begin until he has documented that adequate anticoagulation exists. The surgeon must request that the perfusionist check the direction of flow in the arterial line by circulating the pump prime through the recirculation shunt. He must observe that all suction lines are aspirating rather than pumping air. The surgeon announces the beginning of cardiopulmonary bypass. The perfusionist must visually confirm that the arterial and venous lines have been unclamped and the recirculation shunt clamped. The importance of each discipline having a basic awareness of what should be happening at a given time and being willing to communicate any irregularity in the sequence of events constitutes a system of checks and balances that is the essence of teamwork and the key to minimal morbidity and mortality.

REFERENCES

1. Kurusz M, Wheeldon DR: Risk containment during cardiopulmonary bypass. Seminars in Thorac and Cardiovasc Surg 1990:2:400–409.

23

You have been asked to operate on a 72-year-old patient with congestive heart failure, ascites, renal insufficiency, and chronic intermittent gastrointestinal bleeding. The patient had undergone coronary artery bypass grafting 13 years previously. Doppler echocardiography reveals florid mitral and tricuspid insufficiency. Cardiac catheterization reveals total obstruction of the left anterior descending, circumflex, and right coronary arteries with a 70% narrowing in the left anterior descending graft, a patent circumflex graft but with a proximal AV circumflex lesion jeopardizing the distal circumflex branches, and closure of the graft to the right coronary artery.

Except for some postoperative oozing, which you attribute to chronic passive congestion of the liver and a low preoperative platelet count, the procedure is uneventful. You bypass the left anterior descending artery and a distal circumflex coronary artery, replace the mitral valve with a porcine bioprosthesis, and perform a tricuspid annuloplasty with a Carpentier annuloplasty ring.

Postoperatively, you cannot understand why the patient remains hypotensive, with a blood pressure in the 90/60 range; a heart rate between 60 and 70; filling pressures of 10 and 45/18 mm Hg in the right atrium and pulmonary artery, respectively; a cardiac index of 3.5 L/min/m^2; and a systemic vascular resistance of 665 dyne/sec/cm^{-5}. He requires a combination of dopamine and norepinephrine bitartate (Levophed) and phentolamine mesylate (Regitine) for circulatory support. A technetium=99m wall motion study reveals a left ventricular ejection fraction of 35% with a hypokinetic right ventricle and no pericardial effusion. Although you extubate the patient on the fourth postoperative day, he remains somnolent, lethargic, and confused.

With his persistently low perfusion pressure, the patient's uremia worsens, and he requires hemodialysis. This is performed with difficulty, and the patient becomes truly dopamine-dependent after the first dialysis on the 15th postoperative day, despite significant elevation of the filling pressures. The cardiac index remains elevated at 3.2 L/min/m^2 and the systemic vascular resistance at 628. The patient remains hypotensive, confused, and inotrope-dependent. You are missing something, but you don't know what it is.

SOLUTION

The relative chronicity of this patient's hemodynamic instability in the presence of adequate cardiac function is puzzling. The patient
has no evidence of transfusion reaction, sepsis,
anemia, hypovolemia, or acidosis. A serum
cortisol level is 30 mcg/dL. You did notice a
lidocaine level of 5.7 mcg/mL on the 8th postoperative day but the symptoms persist long
after you stop the drug.

Searching for clues, you review the original
history and discover that, in the past, the patient had taken levothyroxine. Could he possibly be hypothyroid? On the 16th post-operative day, you arbitrarily start the patient on intravenous levothyroxine, 50 mcg daily, after
obtaining a thyroid panel that returns the following levels: T_3: 29% (normal 25% to 35%); T_4
2.6 mcg/dL (normal 5 to 13 mcg/dL); ad-
justed T4 2.5 mcg/dL (normal 5 to 13 mcg/
dL); thyroid-stimulating hormone (TSH) 19.4
mcU/mL (normal 0 to 3.5 mcU/mL).

The next day, the patient's sensorium is
markedly improved. Two days later, the patient is oriented, responsive, recognizes his
physician by name, and is looking for his
bridge partners. He is virtually off dopamine
with a sustained blood pressure of 110/60 mm
Hg and a pulse of 91. After two more days, he
maintains a blood pressure of 125/74 mm Hg
and has a voracious appetite.

DISCUSSION

Hypothyroidism results in decreased myocardial contractility and stroke volume, caused
by alterations in the sarcoplasmic reticulum,
depression of myosin ATPase activity, and
myxedematous myocardial infiltrates with
diffuse interstitial vacuolations containing
mucopolysaccharides and proteinaceous de-
posits. Associated bradycardia results in decreased cardiac output, increased systemic
vascular resistance , a three-fold increase in
plasma catecholamines compared to euthy-
roid individuals, and a decreased blood and
plasma volume.

This patient's laboratory profile suggested
severe hypothyroidism, and he had been on
levothyroxine in the past. He evinced a dramatic clinical improvement within 3 days of
beginning levothyroxine therapy; however, a
cause-effect relationship with this treatment

cannot be proved. Furthermore, other factors
complicated the clinical presentation. For example, this patient had a *low* systemic vascular
resistance. The patient had received lidocaine,
which is known to depress myocardial
contractilityi and to lower the systemic vascular resistance. However, his peak lidocaine
level was only 5.7 mcg/mL (therapeutic range
5 to 10 mcg/mL), and the patient showed no
improvement for nine days after stopping the
drug. Also, the patient was uremic and had
been started on dialysis 2 days before receiving levothyroxine but remained with a low
systemic vascular resistance and hypotension
despite the subsequent measurement of high
filling pressures. Although the white blood
cell count rose from 11,000 to 19,000 at the time
levothyroxine was begun, there was no fever,
bandemia, or positive cultures to suggest occult sepsis as a cause of the low systemic vascular resistance. Prolonged support with
dopamine has been reported to lower TSH
levels and to induce a state of secondary
hypothyroidism; the TSH level may have been
even higher in this patient in the absence of
this drug.

This patient's apparent response to levothyroxine was seemingly rapid. The peak effect of a single does usually occurs in aout 9
days. Thyroid hormone has been reported to
increase beta receptors in the myocardium,
rendering it more responsive to inotropic
agents, and the experimental administration
of T_3 to primates following cardiopulmonary
bypass has been shown to increase myocardial
adenosine triphosphate levels and to decrease
myocardial lactate levels.

The patient expired 4 months post-opera-
tively from uncontrollable gastrointestinal
bleeding. Post mortem examination revealed
angiodysplasia of the duodenum, an eroded
esophageal varix, and diffuse mild nodular
cirrhosis of the liver with congestive changes.
The thyroid gland weighed 10 g and was atro-
phic with colloid nodules. The adrenal glands
were unremarkable.

The differential diagnosis of lingering postoperative circulatory instability must include
occult sepsis, delayed pericardial tamponade,
abnormal responses to anesthetic agents, seda-
tives and analgesics secondary to impaired
hepatic or renal function, and endocrine disorders such as hypothyroidism and hypo-
adrenalism. The diagnosis of hypothy-roidism

was virtually stumbled upon in this case by stepping back from its complexities for a moment and reviewing the patient's history in search of contributing factors that might have been overlooked in the immediate rush of events. Whether or not the diagnosis of hypothyroidism in this patient had any clinical relevance, whether he would have improved at the time he did without the administration of levothyroxine, are questions that cannot be answered. The importance of the diagnosis in this case is not that it had any relevance to this patient's clinical course at all, but simply that it had been *considered* and not by the patient's internist or cardiologist, but by a member of the *surgical* team with a general awareness of broad categories of disease beyond the confines of his own specialty.

REFERENCES

1. Colucci WS, Braunwald E: Cardiac tumors, cardiac manifestations of systemic diseases, and traumatic cardiac injury, in Petersdorf RG, Adams RD, Braunwald E, Isselbacher KJ, Martin JB, Wilson JD, eds.: *Harrison's Principles of Internal Medicine* 10th edition, McGraw-Hill Book Company, New York: 1983, pages 1454-1458.
2. Preedy JRK, Clements SD, Jr, Delcher HK: Theheart and endocrine diseases, in Hurst JW, Logue RB, Rackley CE, Schlant RC, Sonnenblick EH, Wallace AG, Wenger NK, eds.: *The Heart*, sixth edition, McGraw-Hill Book Company, New York: 1986, pages 1412-1435.
3. Haynes RC Jr, Murad F: Thyroid and antithyroid drugs, in Gilman AG, Goodman LS, Rall TW, Murad F, eds.: The Pharmacologic Basis of Therapeutics, seventh edition, Macmillan Publishing Company, New York : 1985, pages 1389-1411.
4. Murkin JM: Anesthesia and hypothyroidism: a review of thyroxine physiology, pharmacology, and anesthetic implications. Anesthesia and Analgesia 1982:61:371-383.
5. Chu SH, Huang TS, Hsu RB, Wang SS, Wang CJ: Thyroid hormone changes after cardiopulmonary surgery and clinical implications. Ann Thorac Srug 1991:52:791-796.
6. Limas C, Limas CJ: Influence of thyroid status on intracellular distribution of cardiac adrenoceptors: Circ Res 1987:61:824-828.
7. Novitzky D, Human PA, Cooper DKC: Effect of triiodothyronine (T^3) on myocardial high energy phosphates and lactate after ischemia and cardiopulmonary bypass. J Thorac and Cardiovasc Surg 1988:96:600-607.
8. Hoogwerf BJ, Sheeler LR, Licata AA: Endocrine management of the open heart surgical patient. Seminars in Thorac and Cardiovasc Surg 1991:3:75-80

24

A 58-year-old hypertensive patient with a history of a right cerebral hemispheric infarction 7 weeks previously complains of frequent episodes of chest pressure at rest, which are associated with shortness of breath. He is known to have had a myocardial infarction 2 years previously and has a serum cholesterol of 308 ng/dL. A dipyridamole thallium study reveals a small anteroapical infarction and septal ischemia, with fixed hypoperfusion of the inferior wall. Cardiac catheterization reveals left ventricular apical dyskinesis with a left ventricular end-diastolic pressure of 12 mm Hg, a 90% to 95% proximal lesion in the left anterior descending coronary artery, a web at the origin of the diagonal, and a 75% circumflex lesion. A preoperative duplex scan of the carotid arteries is unremarkable. With the blessings of the patient's neurologist, you decide to perform urgent coronary artery bypass grafting.

The initial hemodynamics reveal systemic, right atrial, pulmonary arterial, and pulmonary capillary wedge pressures of 132/78, 12, 27/18, and 13 mm Hg, respectively, with a cardiac index of 2.6 L/min/m^2, a systemic vascular resistance of 1503 dyne/sec/cm^{-5}, and a pulmonary vascular resistance of 143 dyne/sec/cm^{-5}. Following the induction of anesthesia and during cannulation, the pulmonary artery pressure fluctuates between 26 and 70 mm Hg systolic, suggestive of repeated ischemic episodes. You abandon your idea to use the internal thoracic artery as a conduit, cannulate, and construct vein grafts to the left anterior descending, diagonal, and circumflex coronary arteries without incident. When you separate the patient from cardiopulmonary bypass, you observe excellent biventricular contractility. You also observe the pulmonary artery pressure to be 90/56 mm Hg, and the systemic pressure only 75/55 mm Hg! Your fingers confirm by palpation that the pulmonary artery pressure is really elevated. As you resume cardiopulmonary bypass, you rack your brain for a solution.

SOLUTION

Convinced that the numbers are real and that the patient has acute supra-systemic pulmonary hypertension, you load the patient with amrinone lactate and isoproterenol hydrochloride and attempt to terminate bypass once again, but with similar results. This time, however, you notice that the proximal third of the left anterior descending graft has gone into spasm with no palpable pulse distally, suggesting that left ventricular ischemia may be the cause of the pulmonary hypertension. You strip the adventitia of the vein graft, apply topical papaverine, relieve the spasm, and restore pulsatile flow to the distal portion of the graft. Despite what appears to be good left ventricular contractility, you postulate residual subendocardial ischemia and insert an intra-aortic balloon. After this, the pulmonary artery pressure rises even higher, to 110 mm Hg. There is no transmission of the balloon pressure wave to the pulmonary artery tracing, precluding the presence of a patent ductus arteriosus. There is no thrill in the pulmonary outflow tract or anywhere in the left atrium, and an emergency Doppler echocardiogram confirms the absence of a ventricular septal defect, mitral insufficiency or stenosis, or a centrally located pulmonary embolus. The arterial pO_2 is 563 mm Hg and a simultaneous mixed venous O_2 is 39 mm Hg.

Having eliminated any mechanical abnormalities, you wonder whether the patient had a drug or transfusion reaction. The patient had been on cefotaxime preoperatively because of a prior urinary tract infection without any clinical or laboratory evidence of an allergic reaction. He had not yet received protamine sulfate, eliminating the possibility of a pulmonary hypertensive reaction to that drug. He had received 2 units of packed red cells during bypass. Could he have had a transfusion reaction? You request the anesthesiologist to administer a gram of methylprednisolone, 50 mg of diphenhydramine hydrochloride, and 50 mg of ranitidine hydrochloride. Over the next hour you observe a gradual equalization of the pulmonary arterial and systemic pressures. By the time you leave the operating room, the pulmonary artery pressure is 47/21 mm Hg and the systemic pressure is 115 mm Hg, augmented.

DISCUSSION

Before arriving at the therapeutic solution in this case, initial diagnostic efforts were directed at ruling out not only other more common mechanical causes of acute *pre*capillary pulmonary hypertension such as increased pulmonary blood flow resulting from a left to right shunt (ventricular septal defect), and reduction in cross-sectional area of the pulmonary bed (massive pulmonary embolus), but addressed, too, causes of an acute rise in the *post*capillary, or pulmonary venous, bed such as acute mitral insufficiency or ongoing left ventricular ischemia. Neither of these seemed probable because of low left atrial pressure and what appeared to be excellent ventricular contractility, despite the distracting presence of transient spasm of the graft to the left anterior descending coronary artery.

This patient experienced pulmonary hypertension, which in all likelihood involved an acute vasoconstrictive process, probably at the precapillary level, for which no specific etiology could be identified. Studies for a reaction to infused blood were negative. The absence of eosinophilia suggested that an allergic drug response was unlikely. Although metabolic acidosis can cause pulmonary vasoconstriction, it was not a factor in this case. Complement-activated leukocytes sequestered in the pulmonary vasculature produce cytotoxic oxygen free radicals that can destroy vascular endothelium and pneumonocytes, resulting in an adult respiratory distress syndrome. Because the patient was never hypoxemic, however, sequestration of leukocytes or platelets in the pulmonary capillary bed during cardiopulmonary bypass was unlikely.

Acute postoperative pulmonary hypertension following cardiac surgery in infants has been treated with intravenous fentanyl, prostaglandins, proscoline, and, more recently, nifedipine, although its effectiveness as a selective pulmonary dilator is not clear. Leukodepletion with special filters on the arterial and venous sides of the bypass circuit, the pharmacologic prevention of free radical formation, and the scavenging of free radicals, should provide additional means of protecting the pulmonary vascular bed from acute injury.

The working diagnosis was one of exclusion based on a review of the patient's history;

intraoperative physical examination, which by palpation confirmed the correctness of the measured pulmonary artery pressure and documented the absence of thrills in the pulmonary outflow tract and left atrium; and the interpretation of laboratory and echocardiographic data that confirmed the clinical impressions. That the diagnosis upon which the treatment was based emanated from the surgical team illustrates the importance of looking beyond one's own frame of reference, with a general awareness of nonsurgical categories of disease that have nonsurgical solutions.

REFERENCES

1. Lee ME: Pulmonary care in Gray RJ, Matloff JM, eds., *Medical Management of the Cardiac Surgical Patient*, Baltimore: Williams and Wilkins, 1990, pages 254–260.
2. Paraskos JA: Pulmonary heart disease including pulmonary embolism, in Parmley WW, Chatterjee K, eds., *Cardiology*, volume 2, Philadelphia: JB Lippincott Company, 1990, chapter 45.
3. Chatterjee K: Bedside evaluation of the heart: the physical examination, in Parmley WW, Chatterjee K, eds., *Cardiology*, volume 1, Philadelphia: JB Lippincott Company, 1990, chapter 31.
4. Royston D: Blood cell activation. Seminars in Thorac and Cardiovasc Surg 1990:2:341–357.
5. Kirklin JK: Prospects for understanding and eliminating the deleterioius effects of cardiopulmonary Bypass. Ann Thorac Surg 1991:51:29–31.
6. Banod K, Pillai R, Cameron DE, Brawn JD, Winklestein JA, Hutchins GM, Reitz BA, Baumgartner WA: Leukocyte depletion ameliorates free-radical mediated lung injury following cardiopulmonary bypass. Presented at the American Association for Thoracic Surgery, 89th annual meeting, 8–10 May, 1989.
7. Davis D, Russo P: Successful treatment of acute postoperative pulmonary hypertension with nifedipine. Ann Thorac Surg 1992:53:148–150.
8. Lowenstein E, Johnston WE, Lappas DG, D'Ambra MN, Schneider RC, Daggett WM, Akins CW, Philbin DM: Catastrophic pulmonary vasoconstriction associated with protamine reversal of heparin. *Anesthesiology*, 1983: 59:470–473.

25

A 75-year-old patient has been evaluated by his cardiologist because of the recent onset of exertional chest discomfort. Although the symptoms are mild, the patient undergoes a treadmill test, which not only reproduces his symptoms at a low level of activity but is associated with hypotension, 4 mm precordial ST segment depression with a prolonged recovery phase, and frequent premature ventricular contractions. At cardiac catheterization, there is good left ventricular contractility with an ejection fraction of 55%. There is a subtotal obstruction of the left main coronary artery and total obstruction of the right coronary artery that fills distally through left-to-right transseptal collaterals.

The patient has had no major prior illnesses, takes no medications, and has no allergies. Your preoperative evaluation includes a duplex scan of the carotid arteries, which reveals mild plaquing with no flow disturbances in the internal carotid arteries, and a scan of the saphenous veins reveals them to be patent and of a diameter suitable for use as conduits.

At surgery, you perform the routine cannulations, which include a right atrial cannula for the administration of retrograde cardioplegia. You begin cardiopulmonary bypass and place vein grafts to the circumflex and right coronary arteries, then graft the left internal thoracic artery to the midportion of the left anterior descending coronary artery. Separation from bypass is uneventful and the grafts lay perfectly. You place right atrial and right ventricular pacing wires, and leave chest drainage tubes in the left pleural space, the anterior mediastinum, and the posterior pericardium.

Once in the intensive care unit, the patient has normal hemodynamics and blood gases, with virtually no drainage from the chest tubes. You feel virtually blessed that this patient has done so well because 6 months ago you captured two press row tickets in the center of the orchestra section for tonight's performance of "Phantom of the Opera," a phenomenon that has always been sold out a year in advance, and you will not be denied what, after today, you believe to be your just reward.

The auctioneer has just illuminated the restored chandelier from the old Paris Opera House. There is an enormous flash as the fortissimo tones of the overture reverberate through your body. Riveted to your seat, you gaze in astonishment as the chandelier rises swinging and glittering from the stage, suspended, swaying for a moment a few feet above the floor before lurching out over the audience. Surely this chandelier is going to land in your lap! But at the last possible moment, it veers sharply upward to complete its eerie ascent to the rafters of the theatre. Almost immediately, the massive set from Chalumeau's "Hannibal" unfolds, flanking the stage with two massive stone idols 40 feet high. Carlotta has begun her aria when you feel that first tiny vibration at the level of your left hip. But it is not Carlotta's aria you feel. It is your beeper call from the intensive care unit.

Benumbed, you slink out of the theater to the harsh luminescence of a telephone booth where you learn that your patient's blood pressure has suddenly crashed. The nurses tell you that the filling pressures have been low for much of the evening and that the patient has required more than the usual amount of volume replacement. There has been only insignificant drainage from the chest tubes, and the abdomen is not distended. They tell you that a repeat chest roentgenogram looks quite different from the normal postoperative film you had seen a few hours earlier, and that you had better come in right away. You slither back to your seat, clambering over half a row of annoyed patrons, press some taxi money into the hand of your loving wife, trample the patrons a third time, and head for the hospital.

SOLUTION

The magic glow of the evening is quickly replaced by the fluorescent glare of a chest roentgenogram thrust onto a viewbox. There is a white-out of the right pleural space. You can hear some air entry into the right lung and there is no mediastinal shift suggestive of volume loss. You can't believe it, but there certainly appears to be a very large right pleural effusion. Confirmatory evidence is provided by the filling pressures, which are in the 2 to 3 mm Hg range, and by the patient's hematocrit, which is 15%.

At surgery the pericardium is dry. There is not a clot to be seen. All the grafts are patent. You do notice a little pool of blood that keeps welling up from underneath the lower aspect of the right half of the sternum. On closer inspection, you see a tiny pumper in the mediastinal fat ejecting blood with mocking precision directly into a 1 cm hole in the right mediastinal pleura. After ligating the bleeder, you open the pleural space widely and evacuate a lake of warm blood, with which the Phantom could have filled the lagoon in the bowels of the Paris Opera House ten times over, into the cell saver. You inspect the pleural space for other surprises, such as the tip of an intravenous catheter, and examine the visceral pleura for evidence of subpleural hemorrhage caused by an overwedged Swan-Ganz pulmonary artery catheter; finding neither, you place an additional chest tube in the right pleural space, and close the incision.

DISCUSSION

This case illustrates one of those perverse, infuriating, unpredictable, unreportable, anecdotal events that can so easily mar an otherwise uncomplicated procedure, not to mention a once-in-a-lifetime evening. Of course, the offending vessel was not bleeding at the closure of the initial procedure. The hole in the right mediastinal pleura had to have been made during the creation of the T incision in the inferior pericardium and was hidden by the mediastinal fat. It was remarkable that the bleeding vessel could evacuate itself directly into this hole and nowhere else. It was equally remarkable, in the sense of being commendable, that the intensive care unit nurses had the insight to order a chest film to help define a puzzling clinical situation. They had expected to find volume accumulation in the left pleural space, related to the dissection of the left internal thoracic artery, with the assumption that the left pleural tube had clotted, preventing its evacuation. This is a prime example of the teamwork that is necessary for superior results. This case also illustrates the necessity for prompt action based upon the information at hand, incomplete and incomprehensible though it may be, rather than hesitation based on denials that, because you cannot come up with an immediate explanation, it just cannot be.

26

A 45-year-old patient with angina has just undergone cardiac catheterization. There is normal left ventricular function, a subtotal obstruction in the left anterior descending coronary artery beyond the first septal perforator, with trivial lesions in the circumflex and right coronary arteries. Several days later, the patient's cardiologist shows you the angiogram and requests that you and your team provide surgical backup for angioplasty of the left anterior descending lesion whenever it is convenient for you to do so. On the day agreed upon for the procedure, the patient arrives as an "A.M. admit" in the cardiac catheterization laboratory. You read over the patient's chart, introduce yourself just before the patient is to be wheeled into the laboratory, inquire about the patient's medications, allergies, and any significant prior illnesses, perform a brief physical examination of the trunk and extremities, and then reassure her that your team will be standing by, in the unlikely event that the angioplasty is unsuccessful, to perform emergency revascularization.

The cardiologists reconfirm the presence of the left anterior descending lesion, insert the guiding catheter and guide wire, and prepare for the first balloon inflation. As they inflate the balloon slowly to 6 atmospheres, a messenger from the record room brings the patient's chart from her previous admission. As you read through it, you are stunned to learn from the referring internist's history that several years previously, the patient had undergone bilateral saphenous vein strippings for varices! What are you going to use as a conduit if the patient becomes unstable, transformed from an elective revascularization into a surgical emergency?

SOLUTION

The solution to this case is that it is better to be lucky than good. You grip the seat of your chair, praying to all the deities of human skill and technology that the cardiologists get through this one without a catastrophe. You can't walk in there and tell them to stop since they are now well into the second dilation. Your only backup is the bailout catheter and the intra-aortic balloon pump. Your institution does not have a percutaneous cardiopulmonary support system. The minutes seem as endless to you as they seem for the patient, but, finally, you see the videotape and hear the cardiologists exclaim to the patient what a great result they have obtained. They thank you with a wave and a wink through the lead-impregnated glass, and you crawl away, a little greyer and a little wiser, armed with fresh ammunition for the next cardiology committee meeting.

DISCUSSION

The absence of a rapidly available conduit under conditions of hemodynamic instability could have been disastrous for this patient. The internal thoracic artery is a fragile structure and does not lend itself kindly to rapid separation from the chest wall. Small tears at the junction of its branches with the main lumen can result in occlusive localized hematomas or long spiraling dissections that will be undetected because of the fat covering the pedicle. Even in the absence of such potential flow-limiting injuries, the internal thoracic artery may not provide adequate flow in the immediate postoperative period to support an ischemic segment of the failing ventricle.

In a patient with no greater saphenous veins, pre-procedural planning should include an evaluation for the procurement of conduits from alternative sources such as the cephalic, basilic, or lesser saphenous veins.

Should these conduits not be available, arrangements to procure cryopreserved saphenous vein allografts should be made. These grafts must be matched to the patient by blood type in advance and are stored in liquid nitrogen at -196°C until thawed for use at the time of surgery.

The essential problem in this case was that the surgeon made a therapeutic decision to provide surgical backup for coronary angioplasty based solely upon the angiographic findings, after the patient had been discharged from the hospital. The surgeon never had the opportunity to review the internist's original work-up, and the cardiologist and the patient neglected to mention the vein strippings. A careful reexamination of the patient's lower extremities after the angioplasty revealed the scars to be virtually invisible, easily missed during a cursory examination.

Early morning admissions for complex procedures may be effective for cost-containment purposes but can be fraught with danger. Invariably, some portion of the pre-procedural evaluation fails to be done in time. The history and physical may arrive late and conceal important information about the patient from consultants whose first contact with the patient may have been the morning of admission. Laboratory work, if not done as an outpatient, may be incomplete and unavailable at the time of the procedure. If the anesthesiologist has had any contact with the patient at all, it may only have been by telephone the night before.

These considerations presuppose that any patient that is accepted for surgical backup is potentially a surgical patient and must be prepared in a similar manner. If necessary, the surgeon must create the conditions by which he can interrogate and examine the patient under relaxed conditions so that provisions may be made to deal with contingencies such as the one described in this case.

Lagniappe

You have been asked to perform a reoperation for coronary artery disease. The saphenous vein has been previously harvested from the right lower extremity from the groin to the ankle. You are unable to assess the size or patency of the left saphenous vein from your physical examination and order an ultrasonic duplex scan to provide this information. The study demonstrates the vein to be patent but with a maximum diameter of 2 mm at the upper thigh level, with a progressive diminution in size more distally. The lesser saphenous veins are equally unsatisfactory. Your examination does reveal bilateral cephalic veins of appropriate quality and size. Knowing this, and with your planned use of the left internal thoracic artery, you are able to decide in advance of surgery which conduit you will use for each coronary artery bypass graft.

The ultrasonic scan provides accurate information about the size and patency of the saphenous veins. It is no longer necessary to make exploratory incisions in the leg to search for the best vein segments. The ability to know in advance where the best vein segments are prevents unnecessary incisions in extremities that frequently are served by a severely compromised arterial blood supply and are at great risk for impaired wound healing and infection, especially in the elderly and in diabetics; the technology should be employed routinely in all patients undergoing coronary artery bypass grafting. Use of the ultrasonic scan in this case enabled the harvesting of the arm veins first with the arms conveniently abducted. Once these incisions were closed, the arms were replaced at the patient's side and the patient prepped in the usual manner for the remainder of the procedure.

REFERENCES

1. Strandness DE Jr: Doppler methods for analysis of arterial and venous disorders, in Hurst JW, Rackley CE, Schlant RC, Sonnenblick EH, Wallace AG, Wenger NK, eds.: *The Heart*, sixth edition. New York: McGraw-Hill Book Company, 1986 pages 1974–1977.
2. DeLaria GA, Hunter JA, Goldin MD, Serry C, Javid H, Najafi H: Leg wound complications associated with coronary revascularization. J Thorac Cardiovasc Surg 1981:81:403–407.

27

You have been asked to evaluate a 73-year-old hypertensive patient who has been admitted to your institution for evaluation of coronary artery disease. He enters the hospital with the recent onset of what appears to be angina pectoris and undergoes coronary arteriography, which reveals severe triple vessel coronary artery disease with good left ventricular function. There have been no electrocardiographic changes or any rise in the cardiac enzymes. As you interview the patient, however, your sixth sense alerts you that this may not be such a straightforward situation. The patient repeatedly describes his current pain as non-exertional and localized more in the epigastrium and left upper quadrant. Indeed, there is some mild tenderness in the upper abdominal area. As you review his laboratory data for the past few days, you notice a progressive decrease in the hematocrit, from an initial level of 40% to its current level of 23%.

SOLUTION

Your suggestion is that the patient be evaluated by a general surgeon to determine whether or not there is any connection between the drop in hematocrit and the abdominal symptoms. The surgeon's evaluation reveals no evidence of upper or lower gastrointestinal bleeding, but an abdominal roentgenogram reveals a calcified mass in the epigastrium, which an ultrasound examination confirms to be a large aneurysm of the splenic artery for which abdominal exploration is performed.

DISCUSSION

The association of coronary artery disease with aneurysmal disease of the abdominal aorta and its branches, peripheral vascular disease, and carotid artery disease is well known and, if unrecognized or left untreated, is a significant cause of mortality in the late postoperative period. It has further been shown that coronary artery bypass grafting significantly improves late survival after various peripheral vascular procedures.

Whether or not coronary artery and peripheral vascular procedures should be performed as sequential or simultaneous procedures is a function of the relative acuity of the two disorders should they become of clinical significance at the same time. In the present case, it is unclear whether this patient really had angina, induced perhaps by the anemia that resulted from a rupturing splenic artery aneurysm, or whether all the symptoms resulted from the aneurysm itself. The approach in this case was to recommend prompt treatment of the aneurysm with appropriate hemodynamic monitoring, to be followed by coronary artery bypass grafting under elective circumstances during the same admission. Had the aneurysm been discovered as an incidental finding in a patient with known operable coronary artery disease, then coronary bypass surgery followed by immediate resection of the aneurysm would have been appropriate. To have operated on this patient's coronary artery disease without having searched for the cause of this patient's anemia would have resulted in profound occult intra-abdominal bleeding with hemodynamic instability. Even if discovered in time, abdominal exploration would have been performed under adverse circumstances, necessitated massive infusion of blood and blood products, and significantly compromised this patient's chances of survival.

REFERENCES

1. Dalen JE: Diseases of the aorta, in Petersdorf RG, Adams RD, Braunwald E, Isselbacher KJ, Martin JB, Wilson JD, eds. *Harrison's Principles of Internal Medicine*, tenth edition. New York: McGraw-Hill Book Company tenth edition, 1983, pages 1488–1491.
2. Diehl JT, Cali RF, Hertzer NR, Beven EG: Complications of abdominal aortic reconstruction. Ann Surg 1983:197:49–56.
3. Cosgrove DM, Loop FD, Lytle BW: Determinants of 10-year survival after primary revascularization. Ann Surg 1985:202:480–490.
4. Carrel T, Niederhauser U, Pasic M, Gallino A, von Segesser L, Turina M: Simultaneous revascularization for critical coronary and peripheral vascular ischemia. Ann Thorac Surg 1991:52:805–809.

28

A 75-year-old patient was transferred from another institution with chills and fever. Eight years previously, a permanent endocardial pacemaker had been implanted to treat symptomatic complete heart block but had to be removed several months later because of erosion of the pulse generator through the skin. The pacing lead could not be removed and had been left in place. A new pacing system was inserted on the opposite side, but the patient was left with a sinus tract that had been intermittently draining in the right supraclavicular fossa for the previous 7 years. *Staphylococcus aureus* was cultured from both the blood and the sinus tract and the patient was treated with antibiotics for about 3 weeks on the medical service with persistent intermittent fever and an episode of gastrointestinal bleeding, thought to have resulted from antibiotic-induced colitis. You have been consulted to remedy this situation. When you first see the patient, you find a 2.5 cm diameter ulcer in the supraclavicular fossa, perhaps made larger by the hemostat that had been placed on the lead several weeks previously in an attempt to keep it on continuous traction.

SOLUTION

Because of this patient's age and his recent history of gastrointestinal bleeding, you decide not to remove this entrapped lead using cardiopulmonary bypass; instead, you attach a 3 pound weight to the lead using an orthopedic traction system, hoping to weaken the fibrous sheath around the lead enough to permit its extraction. You retire for the evening and so does the patient. Eleven hours later you receive an anguished call from the patient's nurse who tells you that just moments ago, at 3 A.M., there had been a terrible crash in room 725, as though the patient had suddenly fallen out of bed. The nurses had rushed into the room to find the patient sitting up, wild-eyed, ramrod straight in his bed, the weight with its line and the lead quivering on the floor in a tiny shimmering pool of dark red blood. Reassured by the nurse that the patient was still in a vertical position with a stable blood pressure and in no apparent distress, you dash to the hospital to witness this miracle of medical science with your own eyes. You recoil in horror when attached to the electrode you see what could only be a piece of tricuspid valve leaflet with several chordae tendinae attached to the remnants of a fibrous sheath surrounding the electrode tip. Although the patient made an uneventful recovery from this debacle, it left you thinking that there must be a better way.

DISCUSSION

The most frequent indication for removal of a pacemaker lead is infection. Failure to remove an infected lead has been associated with a mortality rate as high as 25% and leads to the sequellae of septicemia, endocarditis, and septic embolization. The currently available methods of lead extraction include the traction technique, as demonstrated in this case, and removal under direct vision during cardiopulmonary bypass. The traction method is most successful when used to remove leads that have been in place for less than one year, or for the removal of atrial leads, since the fibrous sheath that invariably forms around the lead in these circumstances is less dense. Complications of the traction method, in addition to the one illustrated by this example, include avulsion of the right ventricular wall, transsection of the superior vena cava, lethal hemopericardium, and arrhythmias.

On occasion, cardiopulmonary bypass must be employed to allow dissection of an entrapped lead from the superior vena cava, the right ventricular endocardium, and tricuspid valve under direct vision. Even under these circumstances, the procedure may be difficult. Chronic thrombosis of the superior or inferior vena cava may resist the most diligent efforts at removal. Adhesions to the tricuspid valve and its chordae tendinae are the rule rather than the exception. Exuberant fibrous reaction to a lead associated with supravalvular, valvular, and infra-valvular tricuspid stenosis has been reported that necessitated replacement of the tricuspid valve. The supravalvular stenosis was thought to have resulted from a right atrial thrombus occuring shortly after implantation, with subsequent organization and recanalization. The valvular and subvalvular stenoses were believed to have originated from the trauma of multiple lead replacements and the constant motion of a redundant atrial lead that abutted the valve, as well as the ventricular lead that passed across the valve, inciting the development of a fibrous sheath that enveloped and fused the chordae tendinae.

If cardiotomy is selected as a therapeutic modality in a patient more than 40 years of age, consideration must be given to evaluating the patient for coronary artery disease before the procedure and for possible coronary artery bypass surgery at the same time. A more conservative approach was selected for the present patient in this example because of his age and his history of gastrointestinal bleeding.

Recently, a technique of intravascular traction and countertraction has been described, which involves sliding a telescoping sheath over the entrapped lead and forcing it down the body of the lead while creating tension on the lead, detaching and/or dilating the fibrous sheath that encases the lead. This method has been successful in removing 226 leads from 124 patients with no mortality and minimum morbidity.

REFERENCES

1. Rettig G, Doenecke P, Sen S, Volkmer I, Bette L: Complications with retained transvenous pacemaker electrodes. Am Heart J 1979:98:587–594.
2. Lee ME, Chaux A, Matloff JM: Avulsion of a tricuspid valve leaflet during traction on an infected, entrapped endocardial pacemaker electrode. J Thorac Cardiovasc Surg 1977: 74:433– 435.
3. Lee ME, Chaux A: Unusual complications of endocardial pacing. J Thorac Cardiovasc Surg 1980:80:934–940.
4. Byrd CL, Schwartz SJ, Hedin N: Intravascular techniques for extraction of permanent pacemaker leads. J Thorac Cardiovasc Surg 1991:101:989–997.

29

A 58-year-old patient enters the hospital because of shortness of breath. Three days following admission, she requires endotracheal intubation for progressive respiratory insufficiency thought to have resulted from pneumonia or acute respiratory distress syndrome (ARDS). All cultures are negative, however, and a rise in the white blood cell count is thought to have resulted from steroid administration for ARDS. A cardiology consultant recommends insertion of a Swan-Ganz pulmonary artery catheter. Hemodynamic monitoring reveals a pulmonary artery pressure of 88/40 mm Hg, a pulmonary capillary wedge pressure of 35 to 40 mm Hg, and a cardiac index of 1.5 L/min/m². Doppler echocardiography reveals significant mitral stenosis and insufficiency confirmed by cardiac catheterization.

At operation, you identify a "fish mouth" rheumatic mitral valve with a 1 cm eccentric opening: fused commissures; and rigid, thickened leaflets, and replace it with a porcine bioprosthesis.

To de-air the heart, you render the mitral prosthesis incompetent by passing a vent across it into the left ventricle, close the atrium, place the patient in the head-down position, activate the aortic root vent, and release the aortic crossclamp. The heart begins to beat spontaneously. You tell the perfusionist you are restricting the flow to the oxygenator and disconnect the left ventricular vent as the anesthesiologist inflates the lungs and the heart begins to eject. You place the patient in the left lateral decubitus position, elevate the head, vigorously ballotte the heart, and invert the left atrial appendage. As you withdraw the vent, you turn the patient to the right lateral decubitus position to ensure de-airing of the right pulmonary veins, and complete the closure of the left atrial suture line. You do not elevate and vent the left ventricular apex directly so as not to incur the risk of a tear in the atrioventricular groove, which is tethered by the valve prosthesis. Your eye then catches an appalling sight; the presence of air in the proximal 2 cm of the aortic root vent. Inexplicably, the root vent has been shut off, and you stand there with no idea whether any air has entered the brachicephalic vessels and the cerebral circulation.

SOLUTION

As you reactivate the root vent and place the patient in deep Trendelenburg position, you decide to retroperfuse the cerebral circulation. You request the perfusionist to attach a length of ¼" tubing to the auxiliary arterial perfusion port of the oxygenator and place a ¼" to ⅜" connector on this tubing as your perfusionist fills it with blood. You then place a snare around the superior vena cava, clamp the arterial and venous lines, connect the auxiliary perfusion line to the superior vena cava cannula, and perfuse the superior vena cava with a flow rate between 200 to 400 cc/min for 2 to 3 min, with the aortic root vent maximally aspirating the retrograde flow. After back bleeding through the aortic cannula to remove any air bubbles that may have entered its tip, you then resume full systemic perfusion and complete rewarming. The patient awakens in the postoperative period with no gross neurologic deficits.

DISCUSSION

Uncertainty regarding the extent of cerebral embolism, if any, prompted the approach taken in this case. The presence of a cannula in the superior vena cava facilitated institution of the retroperfusion. If a two-stage venous cannula had been in place, the retroperfusion could have been performed using a perfusion catheter inserted through a purse-string suture directly in the superior vena cava or in the innominate vein, with snaring or clamping of the superior vena cava below the catheter. In the presence of massive air embolism, retroperfusion of 1 to 2 L/min for 1 or 2 min, with removal of the aortic perfusion cannula to allow full egress of foam from the ascending aorta, has been recommended and allowed full neurologic recovery. As the amount of air embolism was thought to be small because some aortic root venting had occurred coincident with the release of the aortic crossclamp, such a dramatic observation was not possible in this case.

Although the management of this case may be criticized because of the relatively low retroperfusion rate and failure to remove the aortic cannula at the time of retroperfusion, some benefit may have been achieved because of the active suction applied to the ascending aorta during the retroperfusion through the arterial line prior to reinitiating cardiopulmonary bypass.

The monitoring of suspected air embolism may be facilitated by transesophageal echocardiography to document the presence or absence of intracardiac air and by ophthalmologic evaluation of the retinal arteries where air emboli may be observed. Cerebral venous retroperfusion can be accomplished readily and without difficulty and should be employed without hesitation if air embolism is a serious consideration.

REFERENCES

1. Mills NL, Ochsner JL: Massive air embolism during cardiopulmonary bypass: causes, prevention, and management. J Thorac Cardiovasc Surg 1980:80:708–717.

30

A 59-year-old patient underwent implantation of a porcine bioprosthesis 13 years previously because of aortic insufficiency secondary to *α-Streptococcus* endocarditis. He enters the hospital because of congestive heart failure and a new murmur of aortic insufficiency. Cardiac catheterization reveals 4+ aortic insufficiency with a left ventricular end-diastolic pressure of 37 mm Hg, excellent left ventricular contractility, and normal coronary arteries.

At surgery, you identify what appears to be a 27 mm porcine bioprosthesis at the root of a normal size aorta. One of its three leaflets has detached completely from its commissures and is connected tenuously only at the base. Because there is significant tissue ingrowth onto the sewing ring, it is not possible to identify the annular sutures, and you begin to incise over where you expect the sewing ring to be, slowly advancing out to its edge. Using a fine clamp, you are able to separate the sewing ring from its insertion site at one location on the annulus. Having established this plane of cleavage, you grasp the sewing ring itself, gently rotating the valve as you continue around the annulus, staying as close to the sewing ring as possible, and complete the excision.

You are aghast to see the gaping chasm that remains at the level of the sewing ring: 4 mm deep and 4 mm wide. Furthermore, the wall of the aorta ends abruptly, just below the ostia of the left and right coronary arteries, with no direct continuity to the tissue at the aortic root, and maintains this appearance around the entire annulus. This has every appearance of an aorto-ventricular discontinuity, and, as you confront that sinking feeling, you know you must nonetheless formulate and carry out a plan of action.

SOLUTION

You notice that the tissue supporting the gap between the cut edges of the aorta is relatively soft. You pass the first silastic-bolstered mattress suture initially through the superior and then the inferior edges of the defect and observe that it is possible to achieve apposition of the edges without significant tension. You complete the placement of all the annular sutures in a similar supra-annular position, noticing that one bolster, of necessity, is precisely at the orifice of the left main coronary artery. You then pass the sutures through the sewing ring of a 21 mm St. Jude bileaflet prosthesis, the sewing ring acting as a continuous pledget for the inferior aspect of the defect, and lower it into place with its pivot guards perpendicular to the interventricular septum, satisfied that the gap has been obliterated completely.

You accomplish easy separation of the patient from cardiopulmonary bypass. The postoperative course is complicated by low-grade fever, pneumonitis, mild congestive heart failure, and complete heart block that persists throughout this period. Sequential transesophageal Doppler echocardiograms, performed about two weeks apart, reveal 2+ mitral insufficiency that improves between the two examinations. After implantation of a permanent rate-responsive dual-chamber pacemaker, you are relieved to discharge the patient in satisfactory condition.

DISCUSSION

Given the substantial difference in size between the excised porcine bioprosthesis and the new mechanical prosthesis, the original implantation appeared to have been driven by the goal to insert as large a valve as possible so as to avoid the transvalvular gradients inherent in the design of porcine bioprostheses with annular diameters of 23 mm or less. The risks of doing this in the aortic annulus include disruption of the annulus caused by forceful seating of the valve; incomplete seating of the prosthesis, which can result in impingement of the sewing ring on one or both coronary ostia; and gradual erosion of the sewing ring into the wall of the aorta. It seems likely that the latter two

mechanisms were responsible for the line of resection of the valve being only 2 mm below the orifice of the left main coronary artery, and for the deep indentation into the aortic wall, resulting in discontinuity of the intima and probably the media of the aortic root. The fact that a Hancock bioprosthesis was used, with its rigid annulus, perpetuated the tendency for this erosion into the aortic wall to progress. Had a Carpentier-Edwards valve been used, with its more flexible ring, the erosion may have progressed to a lesser extent, but earlier valve failure may have occurred owing to a distorted geometry of leaflet opening and closure.

Given the limited durability of tissue valves, one might question why a porcine bioprosthesis was chosen for a patient who was 46 years old at the time of implantation. The reasons probably included the desire to avoid anticoagulation and an incomplete understanding of the long-term fate of these valves. A recent review of the long-term follow-up of Hancock valves revealed a freedom from structural failure of only 38± 6% after 16 years in the aortic position and 18± 5% after 18 years in the mitral position. A 15 year follow-up of the Carpentier-Edwards standard porcine bioprosthesis revealed a freedom from structural valve deterioration of 71% in the aortic position and 41% in the mitral position. Both series demonstrate accelerated deterioration of these bioprostheses after 10 years. There appeared to be no indication for an annulus-enlarging procedure, such as the Nicks, Manouguian, or Nunez procedures in this patient as the St. Jude prosthesis provides excellent hemodynamics even in the smaller sizes.

Annular suture placement was with the bolsters in the supra-annular position to avoid an excess of potentially thrombogenic material on the inflow side of the valve. This also eliminated the risk of a bolster lost in the ventricle should a suture have broken near the end of the tying process. Fortunately, the tissues were pliable enough that a tension-free repair was possible using the supra-annular approach.

Since there is fibrous continuity between the aortic annulus and the anterior leaflet of the mitral valve, the repair, which essentially involved a resuspension of the anterior mitral leaflet, must have reduced its effective surface area enough that its edge was unable to coapt completely with the posterior leaflet and resulted in a small degree of mitral insufficiency. This has not only been well tolerated but appears to have improved with the passage of time.

The heart block in this patient must have resulted from a suture that passed through the bundle of His that runs beneath the commissure between the noncoronary and right coronary cusps and extends about halfway along the right coronary cusp. To be certain that edema was not the cause of the heart block, the permanent pacemaker was not implanted until the 25th postoperative day.

Aorto-ventricular discontinuity that results from annular abscesses associated with acute endocarditis can be treated by debridement and direct suture closure of a small cavity with orthotopic valve replacement, or pericardial or Dacron patch closure of a large cavity with orthotopic valve replacement. Infection of a prosthetic valve may involve the entire annulus, in which case a cryopreserved aortic homograft valve and segment of aorta, with reimplantation of the coronary arteries, may be employed; or translocation of a new prosthesis more distally in the ascending aorta with aorto-coronary saphenous vein bypass grafts placed distal to the valve.

REFERENCES

1. Oyer PE, Stinson EB, Reitz BA, Miller DC, Rossiter SJ, Shumway NE: Long-term evaluation of the porcine xenograft bioprosthesis. J Thorac Cardiovasc Surg 1979:78:343–350.
2. Bortolotti U, Milano A, Mazzucco A, Guerra F, Testolin L, Thiene G, Gallucci V: Extended follow-up of the standard Hancock porcine bioprosthesis. J Cardiac Surg 1991:6(supplement);544–549.
3. Jamieson WRE, Hayden RI, Miyagishima RT, Tutassaura H, Munro AI, Gerein AN, Burr LH, MacNab J, Janusz MT, Chan F, Ling H, Tyers GFO: The Carpentier-Edwards standard porcine bioprosthesis: clinical performance to 15 years. J Cardiac Surg 1991:6(supplement):550–556.
4. Nicks R, Cartmill T, Bernstein L: Hypoplasia of the aortic root: the problem of aortic valve replacement. Thorax 1970:25:339–346.
5. Manouguian S, Seybold-Epting W: Patch enlargement of the aortic valve ring by extending the aortic incision into the anterior leaflet. J Thorac Cardiovasc Surg 1979:78:402–412.
6. Nunez L, Aguado MG, Pinto AG, Larrea SL: Enlargement of the aortic annulus by resecting the commissure between the left and noncoronary cusps. Texas Heart Institute J 1983:10:301–303.
7. David TE, Komeda M, Brofman PR: Surgical management of aortic root abscess. Circulation 1989:80 (Suppl.1):269–274.
8. Reitz BA, Stinson EB, Watson DC, et al.: Translocation of the aortic valve for prosthetic valve endocarditis. J Thorac Cardiovasc Surg 1981:81: 212–218.

31

You have just arrived home after a busy day during which you performed bilateral internal thoracic artery coronary bypass grafting in a 74-year-old patient with poor venous conduits followed almost immediately by an emergency mitral valve re-replacement in a patient who presented with acute pulmonary edema secondary to a thrombosed mechanical prosthesis. The telephone is ringing as you open the door; the emergency room physician on the line informs you that a 38-year-old patient has been examined in the emergency room because of chest pain that had occurred while the patient had been jogging earlier in the day. The electrocardiogram, except for criteria suggestive of left ventricular hypertrophy, was normal, but a chest roentgenogram, a portable film of poor quality and difficult to interpret because of the patient's extremely muscular body habitus, suggested a widened mediastinum. Although apprehensive, the patient is entirely stable with only a mildly elevated blood pressure that is equal in both upper extremities. The emergency room physician requests your evaluation before embarking upon a more aggressive workup.

SOLUTION

When you arrive in the emergency room, you find the situation as described over the telephone, with one exception: upon interviewing the patient, you discover that he is a weight lifter and that prior to jogging, he had bench-pressed 500 pounds and gave a history of using anabolic steroids. Physical examination is unremarkable.

After studying the chest roentgenogram, and armed with this new historical data, you decide to order an aortogram. The aortogram reveals an aortic dissection that has originated in the aortic root and spiraled into the ascending aorta; in addition, there is 3+ to 4+ aortic insufficiency. While waiting for the operating room to receive the patient, you obtain an echocardiogram, which reveals a pericardial effusion.

At surgery, you cannulate the common femoral artery and vein. Upon opening the chest, you find the proximal ascending aorta to be dilated and violaceous; you can actually see the blood circulating subadventitially. The pericardium contains a large amount of blood-tinged fluid. You cannulate the right atrium with a two-stage cannula and connect it to the femoral venous line with a Y connector. After placing a left ventricular vent through the right superior pulmonary vein, you begin cardiopulmonary bypass with the ventricular vent activated to prevent ventricular over-distension. Upon opening the aorta, you find that the dissection originated in the aortic root, extending to the orifices of both coronary arteries, with a reentry point 15 cm distally in the ascending aorta.

After the administration of cardioplegia directly into each coronary artery, you perform a Bentall procedure, employing a valved conduit composed of a 28 mm Dacron graft and a 25 mm St. Jude valve. Prior to implantation, you impregnate the graft with 25% albumin and bake the conduit in an autoclave. Once the conduit has been seated, you implant the coronary ostia into the sides of the graft and perform the distal anastomosis between the graft and the totally divided distal ascending aorta using Teflon strips inside and outside the lumen. Before releasing the aortic crossclamp, you seal all the anastomoses with fibrin glue made from cryoprecipitate, thrombin, and calcium chloride. You are pleased to observe no suture line bleeding or extravasation through the graft, especially since there was no residual aorta with which to cover the graft.

The patient makes an uneventful recovery. He remains alive and well 4 ½ years later although an aortogram performed 25 months following surgery because of vague chest discomfort revealed a small false aneurysm involving the anastomosis of the left main coronary artery to the graft.

DISCUSSION

The key to prompt diagnostic measures and emergency surgery in this patient who appeared stable in the emergency room with questionable mediastinal widening on a portable chest roentgenogram was the information from the patient that he was a weight lifter. The transient fourfold increase in systolic and diastolic pressure that occurs during weight lifting doubtless exaggerated the forces that normally stress the aortic wall. Repetition of this activity weakened the wall and resulted in an intimal tear. Of special interest is a series of ascending aortic dissections, successfully repaired, that occurred in weight lifters, all of which were associated with medial degeneration upon pathological examination.

The etiology of aortic dissection is multifactorial. Long-standing systolic and diastolic hypertension may result in hypoxia of the medial layers of the aorta, which results in impairment of flow through the vasa vasora. This may cause medial necrosis, which then renders the aortic wall more susceptible to disruptive mechanical forces such as shearing, friction, and turbulence. Medial degeneration also appears to be part of the aging process. Elastic tissue fragmentation seems to predominate in aortic dissections that occur in patients less than 40 years of age.

It has been known for many years that the mortality rate of acute ascending aortic dissection exceeds 90% within 6 weeks of the onset of symptoms and that surgical intervention, which can prevent potentially fatal complications, should be performed on an emergency basis. Such complications include acute aortic insufficiency, pericardial tamponade, obstruction of the pulmonary artery, acute compression of the airway, rupture of a saccular aneurysm, myocardial ischemia secondary to obstruction of flow to the coronary arteries, or potentially reversible obstructions of arteries supplying the central nervous system or viscera.

The operative (30-day) survival rate of patients receiving surgical treatment for ascending aortic aneurysm and/or dissection now exceeds 90% and should be associated with a 5 year survival in excess of 60%. The early and late survival is adversely affected by age >65 years, prior surgery for aortic dissection or aneurysm, distal aneurysmal disease, severity of symptoms, and diabetes mellitus. Recent improvement in survival has resulted from the introduction of hypothermic circulatory arrest, autotransfusion, collagen-coated or autoclaved, protein-impregnated grafts, and the employment of no-clamp techniques on the aorta.

The surgical repair in this case incorporated a complete division of the distal ascending aorta prior to its anastomosis to the Dacron graft. In addition, there was not enough aorta to wrap the conduit after its implantation; therefore, an expansile hematoma capable of imparting tension to the coronary anastomoses could not form around the graft. Nevertheless, a false aneurysm developed at the left main anastomosis. This likely resulted from the patient's insistence upon a continued, though modified, program of body building. The incidence of this complication, here demonstrated to occur using the noninclusion technique, can be minimized by suturing a freed-up button of aorta that incorporates the coronary ostia to the graft, especially if the coronary ostia are a centimeter or less above the aortic annulus, or by suturing aortic wall adjacent to the anastomoses to the conduit,

both of which can reduce anastomotic tension. It is also extremely useful to inspect these anastomoses from inside the graft with magnifying loupes to identify potential sources of extravasation and to repair these with interrupted sutures. The operative mortality of repair of false aneurysms following the Bentall procedure has been reported to be as high as 40%, especially if the aneurysm is large, infected, or contiguous with anterior mediastinal structures.

REFERENCES

1. Anagnostopoulos CE:*Acute Aortic Dissections,* Baltimore: University Park Press, 1975.
2. Shennan T: Dissecting aneurysms. Med Res Counc (Great Britain) Spec Rep Ser 193, Code 45-593, 1934.
3. de Virgilio C, Nelson RJ, Milliken J, Snyder R, Chiang F, MacDonald WD, Robertson JM: Ascending aortic dissection in weight lifters with cystic medial degeneration. Ann Thorac Surg 1990:49:638–642.
4. Crawford ES, Svensson LG, Coselli JS, Safi HJ, Hess KR: Surgical treatment of aneurysm and/or dissection of the ascending aorta, transverse aortic arch, and ascending aorta and transverse aortic arch: factors influencing survival in 717 patients. J Thorac Cardiovasc Surg 1989:98:659–674.
5. Kouchoukos NT, Marshall WG Jr, Wedige-Stecher TA: Eleven year experience with composite graft replacement of the ascending aorta and aortic valve. J Thorac and Cardiovasc Surg 1986:92:691–705.
6. Lewis CTP, Cooley DA, Murphy MC, Talledo O, Vega D: Surgical repair of aortic root aneurysms in 280 patients. Ann Thorac Surg 1992:53:38–46.

32

A 53-year-old patient with a 20-year history of abdominal pain, thought to have resulted from peptic ulcer disease and biliary colic, presents with severe epigastric pain radiating to the back. A histamine H_2- receptor blocking agent and metoclopramide hydrochloride are prescribed with incomplete relief. Three days later, after a normal upper gastrointestinal series and abdominal ultrasound, the patient develops exertional dyspnea and, eventually, orthopnea. A chest roentgenogram reveals bilateral lower lobe infiltrates. Because of worsening respiratory symptoms, the patient is admitted to the medical service the following day. She is afebrile but tachypneic. Examination of the chest reveals a few bibasilar rales and a 2/6 systolic ejection murmur. An electrocardiogram reveals a right bundle branch block with nonspecific ST and T wave changes. A repeat chest roentgenogram shows diffuse interstitial markings interpreted as noncardiac pulmonary edema or opportunistic pulmonary disease. The patient is placed on antibiotics, and blood is drawn to assess exposure to mycoplasma and legionella organisms.

By the third hospital day, the patient is clearly in florid pulmonary edema and requires emergency endotracheal intubation. A loud pan-systolic murmur is heard. An echocardiogram reveals significant mitral insufficiency and suggests the presence of a mass attached to the posterior leaflet of the mitral valve. Cardiac catheterization demonstrates 4+ mitral insufficiency, infero-basal akinesis, and total obstruction of the right coronary artery with distal left-to-right collateralization. You are called to assist with the patient's subsequent management.

SOLUTION

There being no contraindication to immediate surgical intervention, you mobilize the operating room. At surgery, you find no evidence of transmural inferior myocardial infarction. There is, however, a complete rupture of the posterolateral papillary muscle. The torn ends are edematous, suggesting that the rupture had been at least partially completed at the onset of the patient's symptoms. You place a saphenous vein graft to the right posterior descending coronary artery and replace the mitral valve with a 25 mm St. Jude prosthesis. You extubate the patient the day following surgery. A furosemide (Lasix) drip is necessary to achieve a prompt reduction in the patient's positive fluid balance and to help reduce her Aa O_2 gradient. Her course is otherwise uneventful, and you are able to discharge the patient on the ninth postoperative day.

DISCUSSION

This case represents not only a missed diagnosis but the trap that all of us blunder into on occasion: the interpretation of a clinical finding solely within the bounds of one's own specialty. The patient's epigastric discomfort was interpreted by the gastroenterologist as a re-currence of the peptic ulcer disease the patient was known to have and not the subendocardial infarction it really was. The pulmonologist interpreted the chest roentgenograms as showing opportunistic lung disease, possible adult respiratory distress syndrome, and not the pulmonary edema of cardiac origin it really was. Once all the chest films had been reviewed, the pattern of pulmonary edema made clear, and even after an initial echocardiogram was finally obtained, which demonstrated mitral insufficiency, appropriate treatment was not instituted until the patient became so ill as to require emergency endotracheal intubation. As documented by sequential physical examinations, the murmur of mitral insufficiency gradually increased in intensity over a 3-day period and did not dominate the clinical presentation until complete rupture of the papillary muscle had occurred.

Clinicians must not be reluctant to think of, and suggest, diagnostic possibilities that are beyond the confines of their spheres of expertise, even if their familiarity with a disorder can be painted only in the broadest terms. This is what is meant by the aphorism that a physician's responsibility is to know as much as possible about the skin and its contents.

33

A 61-year-old patient enters the hospital because of chest pain. On admission, the blood pressure is 90/60 mm Hg and the heart rate 60. An electrocardiogram reveals marked ST segment depression in leads V1 through V4, with good R wave progression. The creatine phosphokinase rises to 2000 international units and the MB fractionation suggests significant myocardial injury. The patient is placed on a heparin drip but experiences recurrent chest pain that is associated with a drop in blood pressure to 75 mm Hg systolic, and a dopamine drip is started. Two years previously, cardiac catheterization had revealed normal left ventricular function, total obstruction of the right coronary artery, and mild disease in the left anterior and circumflex coronary arteries.

At cardiac catheterization, there is impaired left ventricular function and mild mitral insufficiency. There is now a flush occlusion of the circumflex coronary artery, which the cardiologists open by percutaneous transluminal coronary angioplasty. Although the cardiac output is in excess of 4 L/min, this results from tachycardia, the stroke volume calculated to be 39 cc. Because of this, and with a left ventricular end-diastolic pressure of 35 mm Hg, an intra-aortic balloon is inserted into the descending thoracic aorta through the left common femoral artery, and the patient's condition stabilizes.

Several days later, the patient is able to maintain stable hemodynamics on decreased inotropic support and no longer requires intra-aortic balloon counterpulsation. The cardiologist cuts the sutures that hold the balloon in place, turns off the console, withdraws the balloon as far into the sheath as possible, and begins to pull it out. After about 12" of catheter have been withdrawn, it will reveal no more of itself to the light of day. The patient begins to complain of a numb feeling in his left leg, and the cardiologist thinks of just one thing: you.

SOLUTION

Your initial reaction over the telephone is one of skepticism, but rather than exhort your colleague to pull harder, you wisely decide to take a look for yourself. Sure enough, the catheter will not come out, nor can it be reinserted or rotated. It is stuck, and so are you.

In the operating room, you expose the external iliac artery. As you extend the exposure more proximally, you palpate a hard mass that seems cemented in place. After obtaining proximal and distal control of the iliac artery, you perform an arteriotomy and identify the mass as the balloon, filled with what could only be dessicated blood. The intima of the iliac artery is telescoped distal to the balloon and fragmented as well, precluding any possibility that the balloon could ever be withdrawn in the usual manner. You extend the arteriotomy and divide the balloon catheter so that the balloon itself is delivered through the arteriotomy and the catheter through its original insertion site in the common femoral artery. You tack down the intima distally and close the arteriotomy primarily, as well as the original insertion site, with restoration of excellent pedal pulses.

DISCUSSION

Intra-aortic balloon entrapment as described in this patient is a rare complication of balloon counterpulsation. The prerequisite for its occurrence is a small perforation of the balloon caused by damage to the device during insertion or by prolonged exposure of the balloon to a jagged arteriosclerotic plaque. The telltale sign of perforation is the appearance of blood in the shaft of the balloon. If the perforation is large, there will be a large amount of blood in the shaft; if small, the amount of blood may not readily be visible. A small amount of what appeared to be blood had been observed in the shaft of the balloon in this patient about 18 hours before balloon removal but did not result in immediate cessation of counter-pulsation at the time. As a result, during the deflation phases, blood was repeatedly sucked into the balloon and, as time passed, dessicated by the constant infusion of helium, then transformed into a rock-hard mass that precluded its removal by percutaneous techniques. The only means of safe removal was through a generous arteriotomy at surgery. The incidence of balloon perforations has been reduced since the introduction of long introducing sheaths. Once the diagnosis of a perforation has been made, immediate removal is mandatory before the solidification of the blood inside the balloon mandates a surgical approach.

Retrograde dissection of the aorta has been reported during balloon insertion through the femoral artery. In such a circumstance, the passage of the balloon will be difficult and, if awake, the patient will experience intense lower abdominal or back pain and may develop paraplegia. Fluoroscopy will reveal the tip of the balloon not to oscillate freely in the aorta during the inflation-deflation cycle as it ordinarily does; however, satisfactory augmentation may still be achieved. Removal should be accomplished as promptly as possible since balloon entrapment becomes more likely the longer the balloon remains in an intramural position. Because there is a finite risk of aortic rupture when extraction of a balloon in this position is attempted from the groin, preparations should be made for rapid thoracotomy. Should it not be possible to remove the balloon with gentle traction or rotation, thoracotomy and removal through an aortotomy should be the primary approach.

The most common complication of intra-aortic balloon counterpulsation is ischemia of the lower extremity. Should this occur, and the patient continues to require circulatory support, the balloon may be removed and inserted in the other femoral artery, or a femoral-femoral crossover graft may be implanted to provide blood to the affected extremity distal to the balloon insertion site. In the presence of severe aorto-iliac disease, the balloon may be inserted in an antegrade manner through the ascending aorta or through the left axillary artery.

Emboli to the gastrointestinal tract, kidneys, and spinal cord have been caused by disruption of plaques by balloons inserted through the femoral approach; emboli to the spinal arteries have been associated with paraplegia. Balloons inserted through the ascending aorta have caused emboli to the brachiocephalic vessels both during insertion and withdrawal. Possibly, bilateral carotid artery compression during these maneuvers could reduce the risk of this complication.

REFERENCES

1. Milgalter E, Mosseri M, Uretzky G, Romanoff H: Intraaortic balloon entrapment: a complication of balloon perforation. Ann Thorac Surg 1986:42:697–698.
2. Aru GM, King JT Jr, Hovaguimian H, Floten HS, Ahmad A, Starr A: The entrapped balloon: report of a possibly serious complication. J Thorac Cardiovasc Surg 1986:91:146–149.
3. Richenbacher WE, Pierce WS: Management of complications of intraaortic balloon counter-pulsation. in Waldhausen JA and Orringer MB, eds.: *Complications in Cardiothoracic Surgery*, St Louis, MO: Mosby Year Book,1991 pages 97–102.
4. Lee ME: Mechanical support of the circulation, in Gray RJ, Matloff JM, eds.: *Medical Management of the Cardiac Surgical Patient*, Baltimore: Williams and Wilkins, 1990, pages 164–173.

34

_____

The emergency room has called you to see a 20-year-old patient
who had been thrown off his motorcycle during a collision with
an automobile. On admission, the patient was hypotensive and
unresponsive. He had been intubated, a large bore catheter inserted into the left femoral vein, and now maintains a blood pressure of 70 mm Hg systolic. His pupils are equal, approximately
4 mm in diameter. There is a large hematoma in the right side of
the neck and in the supra- and infraclavicular regions. The right
carotid and right radial pulses are absent. Though not to com-
mand, the patient is observed to move all extremities. The right
upper extremity is in a splint because of a fracture in the right
mid humerus. The remainder of the physical examination is
within normal limits. A chest roentgenogram reveals widening of
the superior mediastinum with blunting of the right costophrenic
angle. The lung fields are clear and the cardiac silhouette, normal. How will you proceed?

SOLUTION

You lead a procession that heads directly for the operating room. Almost as soon as the patient is placed on the table, the anesthesiologist informs you that he is having difficulty ventilating the patient and that the inspiratory airway pressure has progressively risen. He changes the endotracheal tube, but there is no improvement. Flexible fiberoptic bronchoscopy reveals that the trachea distal to the tip of the endotracheal tube has been reduced to a slit, doubtless the result of compression by the mediastinal hematoma. An additional line is placed in the left internal jugular vein. General anesthesia is induced as the patient is rapidly prepped and draped.

You decide to expose the common femoral artery and vein first and insert an additional volume infusion line in the right saphenous vein. You are now in a position to institute cardiopulmonary bypass should the patient become impossible to ventilate. You are relieved when the anesthesiologist tells you he can ventilate the patient and that the blood pressure is now stable at 110 mm Hg following additional volume infusion. Using fluoroscopic imaging, you obtain an arteriogram through a catheter introduced into the exposed femoral artery which reveals, as expected, an extravasation in the distribution of the innominate artery.

After an ill-advised attempt to obtain distal control of the common carotid and subclavian arteries through an anterior cervical incision with a planned resection of the medial third of the right clavicle, which results in the onset of brisk bleeding that an assistant controls with pressure in the suprasternal notch, you heparinize the patient and cannulate the femoral vein for autotransfusion. The aspirated blood is suctioned into a cardiotomy reservoir and returned to the patient with a roller pump, there being no cell savers available at the time this case was done. You then open the sternum from below and gently insert the retractor. Almost immediately, you enter the hematoma that has thus far contained the extravasation from the innominate artery. Your busy assistant manages to control the hemorrhage to some degree as you quickly open the pericardium and sneak up on the origin of the innominate artery at the pericardial reflection and clamp it with a vascular clamp.

You divide the innominate vein, clean out the blood and clots, and are able to clamp the innominate artery distally.

At this point you notice that the left internal carotid artery does not originate from the aortic arch but is actually a branch of the proximal innominate artery itself. By applying a small side-biting clamp tangentially to the innominate artery about a centimeter from its origin, some flow through the left internal carotid artery occurs. You can now see a large rent in the anterior wall of the innominate artery just distal to the clamp. You complete the transsection of the innominate artery and debride the edges. You also evacuate the remainder of the blood and clot from the mediastinum, and you can hear the anesthesiologist breathe a sigh of relief as the airway pressure normalizes for the first time and the lungs, which had remained partially inflated to the extent that the heart was lifted out of the pericardium, deflate. You mobilize the internal carotid and subclavian arteries, clamp them, debride the edges of the tear proximally and distally, and perform an end-to-end anastomosis, which restores pulsatile flow to the carotid and subclavian arteries. Prior to closing the incision, you repeat the bronchoscopy and find the trachea to be of normal patency. The patient awakens, neurologically intact, in the intensive care unit and pursues an uneventful course.

DISCUSSION

Blunt injuries to the brachiocephalic vessels most frequently involve the innominate artery but are seen in only 5% of patients who arrive at an emergency facility alive. The mechanisms of injury include sudden and violent deceleration, crush, or traction forces that result in a partial or complete tear with or without thrombotic occlusion, usually near the origin of the innominate artery. The diagnosis in this case was apparent from the physical examination, which demonstrated absent right axillary and common carotid artery pulses associated with a large hematoma in the right supraclavicular fossa and superior mediastinal widening on the chest roentgenogram. Because of persistent hypotension, the patient was transferred to the operating room, without formal aortography in the x-ray department, where a permanently installed C arm was available for fluoroscopic imaging if the clinical situation stabilized. The development of tracheal compression by the mediastinal hematoma became apparent soon after the patient arrived in the operating room, but, fortunately, ventilation was possible without the requirement for cardiopulmonary bypass.

The common femoral artery and vein were exposed initially for several reasons: to permit rapid induction of cardiopulmonary bypass, if necessary; to provide access for rapid reinfusion of shed blood through a saphenous vein cannula; and to permit aortography under controlled circumstances with the patient ready for immediate thoracotomy. Ideally, angiography should be performed in all patients if they are hemodynamically stable so that the precise nature of the lesion may be identified and the appropriate incision chosen. Computerized tomographic scanning is useful for screening purposes only. It cannot provide the kind of information required to formulate a surgical approach precisely. For the injury described in this case, the proper incision is a median sternotomy first, with a right cervical extension, if necessary.

Retraction or division of the innominate vein provides excellent exposure of the innominate artery bifurcation and facilitates distal control. Primary repair with end-to-end anastomosis of the debrided proximal and distal ends of the artery should be performed if the repair can be accomplished without tension; otherwise, a dacron graft interposition, or bypass from the aorta to the distal innominate artery if the proximal stump is too short, should be done.

This patient's left common carotid artery was a branch of the innominate artery; fortunately, there was enough of an innominate stump beyond the left carotid to allow repositioning of the clamp to permit flow through the left carotid and still have enough of a stump for primary repair. Since the patient had been observed to move all extremities in the emergency room at least 30 or 40 min after the accident, in the absence of a right carotid pulse, it was assumed that intracerebral collateralization to the right hemisphere was adequate. Intraoperative observation of back bleeding or measurement of the pressure distal to the right internal carotid artery clamp would have confirmed this assumption. If it had not been possible to reposition the proximal clamp in such a way as to permit flow through the left internal carotid, cardiopulmonary bypass with perfusion of the left internal carotid or deep hypothermia with circulatory arrest would have been necessary to preserve cerebral function.

REFERENCES

1. Mattox KL: Thoracic great vessel injury. Surg Clinics North America 1988:68:693–703.
2. Letsou G, Gertler JP, Baker CC, Hammond G: Blunt innominate injury: a report of three cases. J Trauma 1989:29:104–108.
3. Rosenberg JM, Bredenberg CE, Marvasti MA, Bucknam C, Conti C, Parker FB Jr: Blunt injuries to the aortic arch vessels. Ann Thorac Surg 1989:48:508–513.
4. Ehrenfeld WK, Stoney RJ, Wylie EJ: Relation of carotid stump pressure to safety of carotid artery ligation. Surgery 1983:93:299–305.
5. Kazui T, Inoue N, Yamada O, Komatsu S: Selective cerebral perfusion during operation for aneurysms of the aortic arch: a reassessment. Ann Thorac Surg 1992:53:109–114.

35

A 41-year-old patient enters the hospital for evaluation of the recent onset of chest pain associated with exertion. A treadmill test was positive and the patient scheduled for cardiac catheterization. The angiogram reveals normal left ventricular function. The left anterior descending and circumflex coronary arteries are normal, although the circumflex system is small with tiny obtuse marginal branches. There is, however, a 1.5 cm long 85% narrowing in the proximal portion of a large right coronary artery that the cardiologists wish to dilate. You are asked to review the film and agree to provide surgical backup for the angioplasty, which, at the patient's request, is scheduled for the following week.

The patient returns to the hospital as an "A.M. admit" after a brief workup that includes a duplex scan to assess the presence, size, and patency of the saphenous veins. You and your team stand by with an operating room ready. The patient is placed on the catheterization table and the procedure begins with a cutdown over the right brachial artery through which a 3 mm angioplasty balloon is passed into a guiding catheter, adjacent to the right coronary lesion. The balloon is slowly inflated to 6 atmospheres for 30 s and again to 7 atmospheres for 2 min. Near the end of this inflation, the patient becomes bradycardic and complains of chest pain. The monitor shows ST segment elevation in the inferior leads. The bradycardia is treated with atropine and then with external pacing through multifunction monitoring, defibrillation, and cardioversion electrodes, which had been placed over the right scapula and the apex of the heart prior to the procedure, but it quickly degenerates into ventricular fibrillation. After four attempts at defibrillation, the rhythm is converted to a sinus mechanism.

Repeat angiography demonstrates total occlusion of the right coronary artery about a centimeter beyond the site of the dilation. During subsequent manipulation of the guide wire, the artery fortuitously opens, revealing a spiral dissection involving the entire right coronary artery from its origin to beyond the take-off of the posterior descending branch. The posterior descending branch itself can no longer be seen. The patient remains hemodynamically stable but complains of low grade chest pain. You have suddenly been thrust onto center stage!

SOLUTION

At the moment ventricular fibrillation occurs, you call for the operating room transporters to come to the catheterization laboratory, order the instruments opened, and the oxygenator primed. The cardiologists remove their catheters and close the brachial artery and the skin incision. Before the patient is moved, they insist upon developing the films and obtaining an electrocardiogram. This reveals significant ST segment elevation in the inferior leads. The film adds no new information to what was seen on the videotape. After a quick word to the patient and his wife, you assist with his transfer to the operating room.

On the operating table, the anesthesiologist inserts a central venous line and an arterial line, as shaving and prepping are carried out. During this time, the patient develops ventricular fibrillation on four occasions, despite a bolus of lidocaine and an ongoing lidocaine drip. All four episodes are easily terminated using the external electrodes placed in the catheterization laboratory with no significant interruptions in otherwise routine but accelerated preparations.

Upon opening the pericardium, you see a somewhat distended right ventricle, with akinesis and mottling of the inferior wall in the distribution of the right posterior descending coronary artery; in addition, you identify a hematoma in the wall of the posterolateral branch, which extends beyond the takeoff of the posterior descending coronary artery. Once on cardiopulmonary bypass, you administer cardioplegia by the antegrade and retrograde routes and construct vein grafts to the posterior descending and posterolateral branches. You terminate bypass easily about 3 hours following the initial closure of the right coronary artery. The inferior wall has pinked up, and there appears to be a slight improvement in contractility. You transfer the patient to the cardiac surgery intensive care unit. No further ectopy is observed during the remainder of the patient's hospitalization.

DISCUSSION

Acute myocardial infarction is associated with primary ventricular fibrillation in 8% to 15% of cases and usually occurs within a few hours of the onset of symptoms. Survival with this arrhythmia is about 80% and its recurrence is unusual more than 48 hours beyond the initiating event. Presumably, the risk of ventricular fibrillation is increased the larger the obstructed artery and the greater the territory it subtends. If the ventricular fibrillation occurs in a setting of impaired ventricular function, the survival is only 20%.

Sinus bradycardia occurs most commonly with inferior myocardial infarctions and is thought to result from stimulation of vagal receptors in the posteroinferior wall of the left ventricle. The danger of the slow heart rate is that it facilitates the appearance of ectopic foci and may, by causing low cardiac output, provoke further ischemia and arrhythmias.

Although the incidence of emergency coronary artery bypass grafting following failed coronary angioplasty is only 3% to 5% and increases directly as the number of vessels dilated increases, patients for whom surgical backup has been requested may be classified at higher risk for morbidity and mortality since the lesions chosen for surgical backup, such as a proximal left anterior descending or multivessel disease, are more likely to result in catastrophic consequences to the patient than dilation of a small diagonal or obtuse marginal lesion. Because of these considerations, patients undergoing coronary angioplasty with surgical backup must be prepared for effective stabilization and rapid transport to the operating room. Once there, the time spent initiating electrocardiographic and hemodynamic monitoring and preparation of the skin should be reduced to a minimum to enable the surgery to begin quickly. Time is muscle!

To accomplish this goal requires the basic understanding on the part of the cardiologist that every angioplasty patient requiring surgical backup is a potential surgical candidate for emergency surgery. The cardiologist must, therefore, have some concept of the mechanics of preparation required to initiate a surgical procedure and be able to tailor his procedure to minimize the surgical set-up time. This requires communication between the cardiologist and the cardiac surgeon.

Several factors conspired to delay and increase the risk of surgical intervention in this case. The angiographic approach selected was through a cut-down exposure of the brachial artery (Sones approach). While enabling a satisfactory completion of the procedure and obviating the need for the prolonged postprocedural observation required after the femoral (Judkins) approach, the disadvantages include the following: (1) extra time required for suture repair of the brachial artery and skin incision, (2) possibility of time-consuming thrombectomy or brachial artery angioplasty in the event of arterial occlusion, (3) removal of a line that could be used to monitor arterial pressure, and (4) absence of femoral arterial access for intra-aortic balloon pumping or cardiopulmonary support techniques that may be difficult to obtain in the circumstance of systemic hypotension or cardiopulmonary resuscitation. Conversely, the advantages of a femoral approach include the establishment of arterial and venous access obtained before the procedure begins, which can then be kept in place to enable monitoring, the central administration of cardiotonic and vasoactive drugs en route to the operating room, and to provide ready access for balloon counterpulsation or cardiopulmonary support.

Protocols for the surgical backup of coronary angioplasty should, therefore, include the following: (1) preprocedural consultations by the cardiac surgeon and anesthesiologist; (2) determination of the absence of contraindications to surgical intervention both before and after the procedure; (3) appropriate consent and crossmatching of blood; (4) a preprocedural skin preparation of the chest and extremities with alcohol or another bactericidal detergent to de-fat the skin, allowing a single-stage iodophor skin preparation in the operating room, if necessary, with or without prior shaving; (5) availability of circulatory support devices (intra-aortic balloon pump, cardiopulmonary support systems) in the catheterization laboratory, with personnel available to operate them; (6) preparation of both groins for femoral access; (7) avoidance of the brachial approach; (8) retention of femoral sheaths for monitoring and volume infusion; (9) use of multifunction monitoring, defibrillation, cardioversion, and pacing electrodes, which can be used directly upon arrival in the operating room; and (10) rapid access to an operating room on the same floor as the catheterization laboratory to avoid waiting for, and transport on, elevators. The ideal circumstance would be for physicians to perform angioplasty in a surgical suite that contains cinefluoroscopy equipment.

The key to optimizing the safe performance of any procedure that traverses the boundaries of two specialties is the communication that enables its execution with maximum efficiency.

REFERENCES

1. Gregoratos G: Management of uncomplicated myocardial infarction, in Parmley WW, Chatterjee K, eds.: *Cardiology*, volume 2, Philadelphia: JB Lippincott Company, 1990, chapter 10.
2. Bigger JT Jr, Dresdale RJ, Heissenbuttel RH: Ventricular arrhythmias in ischemic heart disease: mechanism, prevalence, significance and management. Prog Cardiovasc Dis 1977:19:255–300.
3. Adgey AAJ, Allen JD, Geddes JS: Acute phase of myocardial infarction. Lancet 1971:2:501–504.
4. Lawrie DM, Higgins MR, Godman MJ: Ventricular fibrillation complicating myocardial infarction. Lancet 1968:2:523–530.
5. Holmes DR Jr, Holubkov R, Vlietstra RE: Comparison of complications during percutaneous transluminal coronary angioplasty from 1977 to 1981 and from 1985 to 1986: the National Heart, Lung, and Blood Institute percutaneous transluminal coronary angioplasty registry. J Am Coll Cardiol 1988:12:1149–1155.

36

You have performed an uneventful reoperation for recurrent angina in a 75-year-old patient 4 months following his initial coronary revascularization procedure. The reoperation includes grafting of the left internal thoracic artery to the intermediate circumflex coronary artery, the right internal thoracic artery to the right coronary artery, and the cephalic vein to the distal obtuse marginal coronary artery. During the procedure, you enter both pleural spaces, which now communicate with the pericardium. You insert right and left pleural, as well as posterior pericardial and anterior mediastinal chest tubes at the end of the procedure.

In the intensive care unit, you notice a small right pleural air leak. On the second postoperative day, the patient pulls out his right pleural tube, but there is continued egress of air from the anterior mediastinal tube. At this time, the patient develops a fever associated with leukocytosis and a low systemic vascular resistance, and you add a broad spectrum antibiotic to the patient's regimen.

Twenty-four hours later, the patient complains of severe epigastric pain. The morning's routine chest roentgenogram shows a collection of subdiaphragmatic air as well as a small right pneumothorax. Air continues to exit in small-to-moderate amounts from the anterior mediastinal tube. Physical examination reveals exquisite epigastric tenderness, minimal abdominal distension, no guarding, and no rigidity. Bowel sounds are present. A meglumine diatrizoate (Gastrografin) swallow, which outlines the esophagus, stomach, duodenum, and proximal jejunum, reveals no extravasation. The patient continues to appear septic. How will you guide this patient's subsequent management?

SOLUTION

You find the combination of signs (fever, pneumoperitoneum) and symptoms (epigastric tenderness with an otherwise benign abdominal examination) puzzling and elect abdominal exploration. With the assistance of the general surgeons, this is accomplished using a laparoscope. You discover a hematoma in the upper anterior portion of the parietal peritoneum at the site of the posterior pericardial tube, which had been removed previously. This probably accounts for the patient's epigastric tenderness. The anterior mediastinal tube, which still remains, traverses the peritoneum on its way to the pericardium. One of the side holes of the tube is visible in the peritoneal cavity. Clearly, the right pleural air leak has decompressed through the pericardium and into the peritoneal cavity through the exposed side hole. The remainder of the laparoscopic examination reveals no pathology. The mediastinal tube is withdrawn and a new right pleural tube inserted. The remainder of the patient's recovery is uneventful.

DISCUSSION

This patient demonstrated an unusual cause for pneumoperitoneum without peritonitis. The laparoscopic examination was performed to clarify a confusing clinical picture, complicated by the presence of a pneumoperitoneum, with the least risk and discomfort to the patient and to avoid missing a potentially life-threatening abdominal condition.

Air has been reported to pass from the mediastinum to the peritoneum through the diaphragmatic hiatuses or rupture into the peritoneum from the retroperitoneal space. Pneumoperitoneum without peritonitis has been reported to result from pneumatosis cystoides intestinalis, abdominal paracentesis, laparotomy, recently sealed visceral perforation, and irrigation of a wound with hydrogen peroxide. Distension of a hollow viscus and interposition of the hepatic flexure between the dome of the diaphragm and the liver are well-known causes of pseudoperitoneum.

If there is any question about the diagnosis and its etiology, prompt laparoscopic examination of the abdominal cavity can be performed with little risk and a high degree of accuracy. Cholecystectomy, bowel resection, nephrectomy, and inguinal hernia repair can be performed laparoscopically, as well.

The incidence of the acute surgical abdomen following cardiac surgery is about 0.3%. The most common disorders relate to the complications of peptic ulcer disease (bleeding, perforation), cholelithiasis, and reduction in mesenteric blood flow resulting from embolization or conditions of low cardiac output. Other disorders that have occurred in the author's experience include acute appendicitis, incarcerated inguinal hernia, acute hepatic failure in a patient with known chronic active hepatitis, colonic perforation, and rupture of an abdominal aortic aneurysm.

The operative mortality of the acute surgical abdomen following cardiac surgery is 25%. The operative mortality rate increases if the cardiac surgical procedure is an emergency, involves combined procedures (coronary artery bypass grafting in conjunction with valve replacement or aneurysmectomy) with more time spent on cardiopulmonary bypass, or is associated with a complex postoperative course that includes hemorrhage, pericardial tamponade, and mediastinitis. The risks are compounded if they lead to acute renal or pulmonary failure, stroke, sepsis, ileus, or prolonged hypotension. Any delay in the diagnosis and exploration further increases the risk of morbidity and mortality. It will be of interest to learn whether or not the incidence of intra-abdominal catastrophe increases as more cardiac surgery is performed that incorporates continuous warm retrograde cardioplegia in conjunction with normothermic (or mildly hypothermic) total body perfusion. One might predict an increased incidence of ischemic events in organ systems subtended by arteriosclerotic vascular beds if transient reduction of flow occurs in the presence of normothermia.

Probably the best way to screen patients for the likelihood of postoperative abdominal complications is by a careful review of the history that suggests prior disorders of the various organ systems. Biochemical and physiologic assessment of organ function or reserve may suggest that certain preventive measures should be taken to reduce the incidence and risk of complications or that surgery be delayed or deferred altogether.

REFERENCES

1. Rosemurgy AS, McAllister E, Karl RC: The acute surgical abdomen after cardiac surgery involving extracorporeal circulation. Ann Surg 1988:207:323–326.
2. Lucas A, Max MH: Emergency laparotomy immediately after coronary bypass. JAMA 1980: 244:1829–1831.
3. Zerella JT, McCullough JY: Pneumoperitoneum in infants without gastrointestinal perforation. Surgery 1981:89:163–167.
4. Chandler JG, Berk RN, Golden GT: Misleading pneumoperitoneum. SGO 1977:144:163–174.

37

An 85-year-old patient presents with a history of multiple near-syncopal episodes. On admission, she is found to be in complete heart block with a ventricular rate in the low 30s. The patient is taking no cardioactive drugs and has no electrolyte imbalance; her cardiologist requests that you implant a permanent endocardial pacemaker at your earliest convenience. Because of a slow atrial rate, you both believe the patient could benefit from dual chamber pacing and elect to implant a DDD pulse generator.

At surgery, the patient is comfortable in the supine position with a blood pressure of 150/90 mm Hg. She remains in complete heart block. After prepping and draping the upper chest and neck, you anesthetize the line of the proposed skin incision and the site of the pulse generator pocket with a solution of 1% lidocaine to which you have added sodium bicarbonate in a 1:9 ratio to eliminate the burning sensation of the local anesthetic as it infiltrates the skin. You divide the skin and subcutaneous tissue and reach the pectoralis fascia. Using blunt and sharp dissection, you create a pocket to receive the pulse generator. Having placed the patient in a slightly head-down position, you enter the right subclavian vein with a single stick and pass a J wire into the right atrium. You mold a gentle curve into the pacemaker lead introducer, and it negotiates the curve into the superior vena cava with ease. You then pass a tined ventricular lead containing a curved stylet through the introducer into the right atrium and remove the introducer. As you prolapse the body of the lead across the tricuspid valve into the right ventricle there are a few premature ventricular contractions, but you are pleased to see the tip of the lead find its way through the right ventricular outflow tract and into the pulmonary artery. This is going to be an easy one. You exchange the curved stylet for a straight one, which you advance into the lead as you withdraw it from the pulmonary artery, allowing the tip to straighten. With the gentle pressure and "tissue sense" gained from many similar procedures in the past, you nudge the tip of the lead into the apex of the right ventricle. Almost before you can react, you notice that the lead has assumed the shape of a reverse C on the fluoroscopy screen and that it has passed into the subclavian vein virtually to the hilt! You inform the anesthesiologist to be alert for trouble.

SOLUTION

Because you clearly saw premature ventricular contractions and the lead subsequently pass into the pulmonary artery, you know that this is not a matter of entry into the coronary sinus. Just to be sure, you fluoroscope from the lateral projection and document the proximal portion of the lead to be anterior in the right ventricle. The inescapable, unbelievable, conclusion is that the lead has perforated the right ventricular apex and entered the pericardial space. You tell the circulating nurse to set up a new prep tray and to bring in a pericardiocentesis set, as well as a thoracotomy set for a possible sternotomy incision. You request that the anesthesiologist set up a pressure transducer.

Although the patient has remained hemodynamically stable and you believe the risk of pericardial tamponade to be minimal as long as the ventricular lead is left where it is, you elect not to insert an atrial lead, afraid to compound the problem with an atrial perforation. You remove the ventricular lead and withdraw it into the right ventricle. As you do so, the tip engages the trabeculae near the insertion sites of the papillary muscles of the tricuspid valve. Moving quickly, you ascertain that the sensing and pacing thresholds are within acceptable parameters, fix the lead to the pectoralis fascia, and connect it to a ventricular demand pulse generator, which produces screen after screen of ventricular-paced beats as you secure hemostasis and close the subcutaneous tissue and the skin.

As you complete the skin closure, this truly gargantuan patient becomes restless, flopping and heaving about on the table like a beached whale. The anesthesiologist informs you that the blood pressure has fallen to 90/60 mm Hg and begins administering a lot of "OK, OK" anesthesia. There can be no doubt as to what is happening as you tear off the drapes, splash on the povidone iodine (Betadine), attempt to palpate the junction between the xiphoid process and the left costal margin, grab the pericardiocentesis needle and audaciously harpoon this writhing leviathan, hoping that your needle doesn't lacerate the heart or a coronary artery. You aspirate blood and withdraw the needle, leaving behind an 8-inch catheter, which you attach to a pressure line that has been connected to the transducer you

had requested earlier. You exult in the pericardial pressure tracing you see on the monitor and begin aspirating the blood with uninhibited, high-spirited resolve, watching the intrapericardial pressure drop from 15 to 3 mm Hg as the systemic blood pressure rises to its former level, and the patient, with a grunt and a quivering sigh, begins a flesh-shaking snore to re-enter the realm of a lost dream. After draining about 200 cc of blood from the pericardium, you connect the pericardial catheter to a vacuum drainage bottle and observe the patient for the next 24 hours in the intensive care unit. After that time, there being minimal drainage, stable hemodynamics, and no reaccumulation of pericardial fluid as determined by echocardiography, you remove the catheter, and the remainder of the patient's recovery is unremarkable.

DISCUSSION

The implantation of permanent endocardial pacemakers is, ostensibly, a straightforward surgical procedure, yet can be complicated by acute problems that require immediate diagnosis and appropriate action. In this case, the occurrence of pericardial tamponade was anticipated, in the knowledge that the catheter had, without any doubt, entered the right ventricle (based upon the induction of a few premature ventricular contractions and the presence of the lead in the pulmonary artery) and not the coronary sinus.

If one can predict the presence of a bloody pericardial effusion, it is extremely useful to be able to differentiate between blood that has extravasated into the pericardium and blood that comes from within the right ventricle. With the goal being the withdrawal of as much blood as possible in the shortest time, it is comforting to know that the aspirating catheter is in the pericardium and not the right ventricle. This kind of reassurance cannot be provided by pericardiocentesis techniques that rely upon needle-induced electrocardiographic evidence of myocardial injury. Under elective circumstances, in the intensive care unit, or under emergent but anticipated circumstances in the operating room, it is possible to set up a pressure transducer that will unerringly identify the location of a catheter by displaying a pericardial or a right ventricular pressure tracing on the monitor.

The use of stylets to aid in seating pacemaker leads is a common practice. It is probably wise to use the thinnest gauge, most flexible stylet available and to keep it withdrawn a half centimeter from the tip of the lead to provide the maximum lead flexibility during implantation. The perforation in the present case occurred with absolutely no sensation of the lead perforating the myocardium, the only evidence provided by the striking and painfully obvious image of the lead traversing a lazy arc in the pericardial space on the fluoroscopy screen. This occurrence is more likely to happen in a myocardium that has been recently infarcted; in such circumstances, efforts should be made to avoid the right ventricular apex and to locate the lead in the base of the right ventricle, which is rarely infarcted or, using a screw-in lead, to affix it to the interventricular septum or the pulmonary outflow tract.

In some circumstances, specifically in the presence of a tricuspid valve prosthesis, it is either inadvisable or impossible to pass a lead into the right ventricle. If the valve replacement is remote in time, ventricular capture may be achieved with a lead passed into the coronary sinus and down the posterior or anterior descending veins. If appropriate sensing or pacing thresholds cannot be achieved using this method, epicardial leads can be implanted using a subxiphoid approach or through a left anterior thoracotomy. In order to obviate this problem, epicardial leads should be implanted at the time of tricuspid valve replacement.

Another acute problem relating to lead implantation with a similar clinical presentation is tension pneumothorax; however, entry into the subclavian vein with a single stick significantly reduced the likelihood that the patient's dilemma resulted from a pneumothorax caused by a laceration to the apex of the lung. Other less frequent problems of implantation include perforation of the junction of the superior vena cava and the innominate vein with an introducer and cannulation of the subclavian artery with pacing established from the apex of the left ventricle.

It is of critical importance that individuals who implant pacemakers be aware of the rapidity with which patients can find themselves thrust into life-threatening situations during a procedure that is so "simple." Because of this, primary pacemaker implantation should be performed in an operating room with an anesthesiologist in attendance who can deal with the unruly or unstable patient while the surgeon deals with the underlying emergency.

38

You have been asked to perform coronary artery bypass surgery on a 75-year-old patient with impaired left ventricular function, severe distal disease, and limited run-off into the coronary bed. Because of pre-induction ischemia manifested by ST segment changes on the monitor and transient elevations in the pulmonary artery pressure, you insert an intra-aortic balloon pump prior to mediastinotomy. With appropriate counterpulsation and pharmacologic adjustments of the patient's hemodynamics, a degree of stability is achieved that permits harvesting of the saphenous vein and cannulation to proceed in a safe and routine manner. Employing antegrade-retrograde crystalloid cardioplegia with ultrafiltration, you construct grafts to the left anterior descending, diagonal, circumflex, and right coronary arteries and are able to terminate cardiopulmonary bypass with balloon counterpulsation and atrial pacing, without inotropic support.

In the immediate postoperative period, the mediastinal tubes drain about 150 cc/hour. This is associated with a platelet count of 52,000 per mm^3 and a partial thromboplastin time of 106 s. With evidence for a coagulopathy, as well as the fact that the patient had ingested aspirin prior to surgery, you administer fresh frozen plasma and platelets and start positive end-expiratory pressure to help compress the mediastinal structures and potential mediastinal bleeding points. Over the next several hours, the bleeding stops, the hemodynamics remain stable, and you settle in for a good night's sleep.

The telephone jangles the instant your head touches the pillow; of course, it is your faithful nurse in the intensive care unit informing you that your patient's blood pressure has dropped to 70 mm Hg systolic at about the same time that, after several hours of minimal drainage, 300 cc of warm red blood had gushed into the autotransfusion bag. The nurse has started a dopamine drip and is preparing to reinfuse the shed blood, and you decide you had better move fast!

SOLUTION

You request the nurse to call the operating room to mobilize the cardiac surgical team, as well as the blood bank to type and crossmatch the patient for additional units of blood. As you jump into the car, you know that the operating room will call in the heart nurses, cardiac anesthesiologist, and perfusionist who will, at the very least, run the cell saver. When you arrive in the intensive care unit 20 min later, you help prepare for the patient's immediate transfer to the operating room, always a clumsy business, more so tonight because of the ventilator and the balloon pump console. You are not satisfied with the patient's blood pressure response to volume infusion: the monitor shows an atrially paced rate of 90, the intra-aortic balloon is firing on a 1:1 setting, the dopamine is running, but the blood pressure remains in the 80s.

Pushing the ventilator and bed, pulling the balloon console, with a pole of infusion pumps rattling and lurching behind you, your caravan clatters down the hallway, jolted to an occasional abrupt stop as the bed hits a door jamb, swinging around corners in a massive arc and pinning the anesthesiologist, who loses the bag for a breath or two, against the wall, finally to enter the ice-cold operating room where the scrub nurse is well on her way to being set up.

You never really notice when the blood pressure disappears. All you know is that the anesthesiologist is telling you there is none. You pull down the bed rail, tear off the dressing and cut through the steristrips as a circulating nurse throws on the povidone iodine (Betadine). You quickly reach the wires, cut them, and insert a retractor. The blood wells up and as you clear away some clot, taking care not to avulse a graft, you despair to find the heart motionless. As you begin cardiac massage, you glance at the pacing spikes on the monitor, dutifully triggering the balloon pump. Fortunately, the heart is full and you are able to generate a blood pressure. After 10 min of massage, the injection of epinephrine and calcium chloride into the apex of the left ventricle, and a single defibrillation, you restore a regular rhythm, a stable blood pressure, and transfer the patient to the operating table. You identify small bleeding points at the proximal and distal anastomoses of the diago-

nal graft and repair them. You return the patient to the intensive care unit in stable condition. After an initial period of ischemic encephalopathy, the patient makes a full recovery and leaves the hospital in satisfactory condition.

DISCUSSION

Bleeding in excess of 10 cc/kg for any hour, or 5 cc/kg for each of the first 3 hours in the postoperative period, is an indication for exploration to rule out a surgical cause. This dictum can be modified by the early identification of a coagulopathy that is amenable to prompt correction with pharmacologic agents or specific blood products such as fresh frozen plasma, specific clotting factors, and platelets. In the present case, a coagulation disorder was not suspected until after the patient had arrived in the intensive care unit, where fresh frozen plasma and platelets were given. This treatment induced clotting but resulted in a multiloculated mass that accumulated in the mediastinum and pericardium and essentially obstructed free drainage through the chest tubes, despite the efforts of the intensive care unit nurses to keep them patent. Had the coagulopathy been suspected in the operating room, the blood products would have been administered there so that their effect could be evaluated and excess clot formation removed with the chest open to prevent a near-catastrophic tamponade. It is always better to spend whatever time is required to secure hemostasis by surgical or medical means at the initial procedure.

When a coagulopathy is treated in the intensive care unit, one must be on constant alert for the development of tamponade; the cessation of bleeding through the chest tubes must never be regarded as the cessation of bleeding, which, as in this case, can continue to fill the pericardium, unable to drain through clot-obstructed tubes. Pericardial tamponade can occur whether or not the pericardium and both pleural spaces remain open. Opening the pleural spaces may, in fact, be disadvantageous, permitting occult blood loss there that is never reflected in the chest tube drainage and may be identified only on the basis of a chest roentgenogram, if the thought occurs to anyone and if the clinical situation permits the time to be spent obtaining it.

Attempts to clear mediastinal tubes using embolectomy catheters may clear the lumen of clot but will not clear the mass of clot enveloping the tubes; furthermore, there is a risk of perforating the heart and introducing infection using this method. A more effective means of pericardial decompression, other than mediastinotomy in the intensive care unit, is removal of the tubes altogether.

Rapid re-entry into the chest of an unstable patient is decidedly facilitated by using a subcuticular suture, and not staples, to close the initial chest incision. If the patient is especially unstable, reoperation may be performed safely in the intensive care unit. This avoids the time lost, risks, and inconvenience of transport to the operating room, but still requires the presence of operating room nurses and availability of a fiberoptic headlight.

The most frequent causes of nonsurgical bleeding include inadequate neutralization of heparin, thrombasthenia related to aspirin ingestion, thrombocytopenia, hyperfibrinolysis, clotting factor deficiencies, and disseminated intravascular coagulation. These disorders are usually treated with fresh frozen plasma and platelets. With regard to pharmacologic agents, the use of desmopressin acetate (DDAVP) is controversial at best, with several series demonstrating no benefit in reducing postoperative hemorrhage and others actually documenting a 30% increase, possibly secondary to a three- to four fold increase in the level of tissue plasminogen activator, which results in a fibrolytic state. Aprotinin is a proteinase inhibitor that has been associated with signifi-

cant reductions in postoperative blood loss. It appears to act by the preservation of adhesive platelet receptors and by the inhibition of kallikrein formation, which is essential in the activation of factor XII and the intrinsic clotting system during cardiopulmonary bypass. The latter mechanism has been associated with decreased requirements for heparin during cardiac surgery. Amicar (epsilon-aminocaproic acid) has been used to treat primary fibrinolysis. If used in error to treat fibrinolysis secondary to disseminated intravascular coagulation, diffuse intravascular thrombosis may result.

REFERENCES

1. Mammen EF, Koets MH, Washington BC, et al.: Hemostasis changes during cardiopulmonary bypass. Semin Thromb Hemost 1985:11:281–292.
2. Kaiser, GC, Naunheim KS, Fiore AC, Harris HH, McBride LR, Pennington G, Barner HB, William VL: Reoperation in the intensive care unit. Ann Thorac Surg 1990:49:903–908.
3. LoCicero J III, Massad M: Any value for desmopressin acetate (DDAVP) in cardiopulmonary bypass operation? (letter to the editor). J Thorac Cardiovasc Surg 1990:99:945
4. van Oeveren W, Harder MP, Roozendaal KJ, Eijsman MD, Wildevuur CRH: Aprotinin protects platelets against the initial effect of cardiopulmonary bypass. J Thorac Cardiovasc Surg 1990:99:788–797.
5. de Smet AAEA, Joen MCN, van Oeveren W, Roozendaal KJ, Harder MP, Eijsman L, Wildevuur CRH: Increased anticoagulation during cardiopulmonary bypass by aprotinin. J Thorac Cardiovasc Surg 1990:100:520–527.

39

This hasn't been a time you care to remember. Not only had your recent evening at the "Phantom of the Opera" been unceremoniously shattered but you can only marvel at the telephone call you receive some days later from the intensive care unit. You had performed a mitral valve replacement for mitral stenosis in an otherwise healthy patient. You would have preferred to replace the valve with preservation of the chordae tendinae and papillary muscles, but owing to thickened, calcified leaflets and fused chordae tendinae, this was not possible. The procedure had been straightforward and you are utterly baffled as to why you find yourself climbing into your car once again at 2 o'clock in the morning to see a patient with deteriorating blood gases and with what the nurse believes to be a massive right pleural effusion on a chest roentgenogram she had ordered. This case had not been a reoperation; you had not knowingly violated the pleural space during the sternotomy or during the lateral extension of the pericardiotomy at the diaphragm; and there had not been any significant drainage from the mediastinal catheters, a drop in hematocrit, or hemodynamic instability to suggest ongoing blood loss.

Upon your arrival in the intensive care unit, you see that the chest film, indeed, shows a large right pleural effusion. The immediate postoperative film had demonstrated clear lung fields. Where had that effusion come from?

SOLUTION

You perform a thoracentesis in the midaxillary line in the fifth intercostal space and easily withdraw a syringe full of clear yellow fluid. You insert a chest tube at the same site and watch 1500 cc of the same fluid rapidly fill the drainage bottle. A repeat chest film demonstrates resolution of the effusion. It also suggests that a central venous line, which had been inserted through the left internal jugular vein, appears to have migrated slightly to the right. Could its tip be in the right pleural space? You add some methylene blue to the bottle of 5% albumin that is running through the line and soon observe that the drainage from the pleural space acquires a greenish hue. Having confirmed your suspicion, you elect to return the patient to the operating room where you observe the tip of the central venous line protruding through the junction of the innominate vein with the superior vena cava. As the anesthesiologist slowly withdraws it, you control the puncture site with a suture, return the patient to the intensive care unit, and return to your thoughts and your bed, thoroughly convinced that there must be a phantom haunting the operating room as well.

DISCUSSION

It is distracting during a cardiac surgical procedure to experience problems with the cannulations required for monitoring and the conduct of cardiopulmonary bypass. The insertion of the central venous line through the left internal jugular vein represented a departure from the usual insertion site through the right internal jugular vein. Central venous lines are usually inserted through the right internal jugular vein because of the relatively straight course provided to access the superior vena cava and the right side of the heart. The left side had been used in this case because of anticipated difficulties passing lines through or near scar tissue associated with this patient's prior right carotid endarterectomy. Although blood had been easily aspirated through the catheter immediately upon insertion, the tip of the catheter had not negotiated the junction between the innominate vein and the superior vena cava and over a period of hours had migrated through the wall, exposing the tip to the pleural space. Once the diagnosis had been confirmed, surgical exploration was elected to directly repair the hole, there being no structures other than the lung able to tamponade the defect with the same degree of reliability as a well-placed suture.

Numerous other complications of cervical central venous cannulation have been described. These include injury to the carotid artery; phrenic or other cervical nerves; and to the thoracic duct, especially on the left side. Unintentional cannulation of a carotid or subclavian artery occurs in about 1% of cases. Penetration with an exploring needle is of no consequence, but cannulation with a central line or a sheath necessitates delay of the intended procedure to prevent catastrophic hemorrhage into a body cavity or along tissue planes during heparinization, which may be fatal if unrecognized, or recognized too late. If the cardiac procedure must be done, prior repair of the puncture site under direct visualization is mandatory.

Air embolism is an ever-present risk from central venous catheterization. In order to reduce this risk, the procedure should be performed with the patient in the head-down position, especially in the presence of a low central venous pressure. Air embolism has been reported to occur with only a guide wire in place but is more frequent during insertion, removal, or damage to a catheter, as well as during the injection of medications with a syringe or the piggybacking of intravenous solutions. In all fairness to the anesthesiologists, the frequent presence of air in the innominate vein upon opening the sternum probably results, in part, from venous air embolism through the sternal marrow upon sternotomy. Robicsek et al. described contrast medium injected into the sternal bone marrow of dogs to appear rapidly in the azygous and hemiazygous systems, then to the superior vena cava and the pulmonary circulation.

In the 20% to 30% of adults that have a patent foramen ovale, especially in the presence of elevated right atrial pressure or in the presence of cyanotic congenital heart disease with right to left shunting, the risk of air embolism extends beyond the symptoms and signs of tachypnea, chest pain, and arterial desaturation to include systemic air embolization.

Other complications of central venous cannulation include creation of an arteriovenous fistula by a catheter that traverses an artery before entering a vein, pneumothorax, hemothorax, and pericardial tamponade, all of which can be associated with the local extravasation of fluids and drugs; and shearing and embolization of the catheter itself, the latter requiring retrieval with ureteral stone baskets or flexible bronchoscopy biopsy forceps to prevent in-situ thrombosis or infection.

REFERENCES

1. Skeehan TM, Thys DM: Monitoring the cardiac surgical patient, in Hensley FA, Martin DM eds.: *The Practice of Cardiac Anesthesia*, Boston: Little Brown and Co., 1990, page 150.
2. Kron IL, Joob AW, Lake CL, Nolan SP: Arch vessel injury during pulmonary artery catheter placement. Ann Thorac Surg 1985:39:223–224.
3. Poterack KA, Aggarwal A: Central venous air embolism without a catheter. Can J Anaesth 1991:38:338–340.
4. Gottdiener JS, Papademetriou V, Notargiacomo A, Park WY, Cutler DJ: Incidence and cardiac effects of systemic venous air embolism: echocardiographic evidence of arterial embolization via noncardiac shunt. Arch Int Med 1988:148:795–800.
5. Presson RG Jr, Kirk KR, Haselby KA, Linehan JH, Zaleski S, Wagner WW Jr. : Fate of air emboli in the pulmonary circulation. J Appl Physiol 1989:67:1898–1902.
6. Robicsek F, Masters TN, Littman L, Born GVR: The embolization of bone wax from sternotomy incisions. Ann Thorac Surg 1981:31:357–359.
7. Thompson T, Evans W: Paradoxical embolism. Quart J Med 1930:23:135–150.
8. McGinn S, White PD: Progress in recognition of congenital heart disease. N Engl J Med 1936: 214:763–768.

40

A 57-year-old patient with a history of coronary artery bypass grafting both 20 and 10 years previously, enters the hospital for cardiac catheterization after recurrent episodes of congestive heart failure. Recent Doppler echocardiography revealed severe mitral insufficiency with mild depression of left ventricular contractility. Catheterization reveals a left ventricular ejection fraction of 45% with florid mitral insufficiency and a left ventricular end diastolic pressure of 35 mm Hg. The right atrial, pulmonary arterial, and pulmonary capillary wedge pressures are 20, 85/44, and 36 mm Hg, respectively. Coronary arteriography reveals total obstruction of the left anterior descending, circumflex, and right coronary arteries. There is a patent left internal thoracic artery graft to the left anterior descending and patent vein grafts to the circumflex and right coronary arteries. The circumflex graft is ectatic with a 75% narrowing but remains unchanged from its appearance on an angiogram that had been performed 3 years previously and supplies a tiny vessel. Following the catheterization, the patient develops florid pulmonary edema and is transferred to the intensive care unit for diuresis and your surgical evaluation.

You concur that an intervention on the mitral valve is indicated. Since this represents the patient's third open-heart procedure, you elect mitral valve replacement rather than risk a less than perfect repair, and select the transvalvular approach to preserve the geometry of what remains of this patient's left ventricular contractility, which, in an unloaded ventricle, generates only a 45% ejection fraction. In order to avoid dissecting out the entire heart from its adhesions and because of the small circumflex, you decide not to regraft it. As you examine the chest roentgenogram, you notice what you perceive to be the greatest risk of the procedure: The internal thoracic graft, as outlined by the clips on its branches, forms a gentle loop that places it directly under the sternum virtually at the midline. To prevent turning this third cardiac procedure into a total rout should this vessel be divided during entry into the chest, you must formulate a plan to protect it and the myocardium it supplies.

SOLUTION

As is a routine for all reoperations, you place external defibrillation pads over the right scapula and the apex of the heart prior to prepping and draping to facilitate defibrillation should the heart fibrillate during sternotomy or before the heart has been divested of its adhesions. You request a ¼" arterial perfusion line from the oxygenator, which is fitted with arterial pressure tubing and a cannula ordinarily used to distend saphenous veins for perfusion of the distal end of the internal thoracic artery graft should it be divided during mediastinal entry.

You expose and cannulate the right common femoral artery and vein with a Y connector on the venous line to supplement the venous return with right atrial cannulas once the heart has been exposed.

Rather than dividing and removing the sternal wires, you untwist them and leave them in place to help limit the depth of penetration of the sternal saw. You separate as much of the superior mediastinal tissue as possible from the underside of the sternum with cautious finger dissection and, with a sigh of relief, accomplish sternal division uneventfully. To avoid the induction of ventricular fibrillation, you do not use the cautery but employ sharp dissection to separate the mediastinal structures from the undersurface of the sternal edges. This allows insertion of a retractor. You cannulate the superior and inferior venae cavae and place a retrograde cardioplegia cannula in the right atrium. You do not expose the aorta as you have not yet identified the internal thoracic artery pedicle.

You must now identify the internal thoracic artery pedicle and encircle it with a vessel loop so that during cardiopulmonary bypass it may be clamped to prevent washout of cardioplegia. You accomplish this by sharp dissection of all the mediastinal fat from the upper left sternum and from the right ventricular outflow tract. The exposure is facilitated by gentle upward traction on the left half of the sternum. You encircle a 4 cm diameter mass of fat that you believe must contain the pedicle and confirm that it does by application of a sterile Doppler transducer that broadcasts vigorous flow. You then dissect out the ascending aorta, insert an aortic root perfusion-venting catheter and begin cardiopulmonary bypass using antegrade-intermittent retrograde cold right atrial crystalloid cardioplegia with ultra-filtration.

The mitral insufficiency resulted from significant prolapse of the anterior leaflet with attenuation of the posterior leaflet. After exclusion of the left atrial appendage with an internal purse-string suture, you accomplish a transvalvular implantation of a St. Jude bileaflet valve and begin to rewarm. Upon release of the aortic crossclamp, the heart begins to beat spontaneously and you begin the de-airing process.

Just as you begin to relax and comment on how well things had progressed to this point, the perfusionist informs you of a sudden dramatic increase in the arterial line pressure, which has necessitated an abrupt reduction in flow. There having been no change in position of the cannula and no kinks or clamps on the line, you suspect that the tip of the cannula has lifted a plaque in the femoral artery, which has resulted in a partial obstruction to flow, or an incipient retrograde dissection. You quickly place a purse-string suture in the ascending aorta, insert an aortic perfusion cannula, and reestablish flow through the aorta. The remainder of the operative course and the patient's recovery are uneventful.

DISCUSSION

Success with a case of this complexity depends upon decision making that encompasses what must be accomplished, what shouldn't be attempted, what is most likely to go wrong, and how to deal with what might go wrong. One must strive for simplicity, retain the ability to change one's plan rapidly if required, and—why not admit it—hope for some good luck. The major goal of this operation was mitral valve replacement without causing damage to the internal thoracic artery graft. The circumflex graft was not redone, not only because of the small size of the circumflex coronary artery, but also because of the risks of potential damage to the internal thoracic artery pedicle, the tethering of the heart by the pedicle rendering it difficult to rotate for exposure of the circumflex, and the necessity to dissect out the entire heart, which would have added the risk of pericardial tamponade in the postoperative period. These concerns were weighed against the risk to the patient of ultimate closure of the circumflex graft, which was regarded as small.

The application of external defibrillation

pads prior to prepping provided the opportunity for effective defibrillation without the necessity for rapid dissection of the heart from its adhesions to apply paddles directly on the epicardium. This, too, would have subjected the pedicle to risk of damage.

The cautery was avoided in the dissection because of its capability to induce ventricular fibrillation during vulnerable periods of the cardiac cycle. If cautery must be used near or on the heart in any cardiac surgical case it should be applied only during the refractory period of the cardiac cycle, as identified by the midportion of the T wave on the surface electrocardiogram, a point at which it is not possible to stimulate the myocardium.

With all the precautions taken before and during this case, an unexpected incipient retrograde dissection occurred in the common femoral artery that required urgent recannulation. If cardiopulmonary bypass had been initiated and the rise in line pressure occurred earlier in the case, before the internal thoracic artery pedicle had been identified and the aorta safely cleared, a more extensive aortic dissection may have occurred and injury to the pedicle resulted either from the aortic dissection or from a hasty attempt to clear the ascending aorta. This would have resulted in the simultaneous confrontation of two potentially lethal problems. It was only good fortune that spared the patient that dilemma.

Afterword

To paraphrase Newton, all of us have stood upon the shoulders of giants to see more clearly the road to our goal: the delivery of optimal health care to our patients. Not always prepared emotionally or by experience to comprehend fully the vistas that stretch before us, buffeted by winds of uncertainty, bad judgment, gross error, and feelings of inadequacy while trying to maintain our balance at these dizzying heights, we discover that the learning process is lengthy, arduous, painful, and, occasionally, lethal. We then perceive that it is advantageous to our sense of accomplishment, and to the survival of our patients, not to make the same mistake twice. Compassion alone is not enough; the world is full of well-meaning people.

The key to achieving the most consistently successful delivery of health care is the acquisition of knowledge and its wise, compassionate, and skillful application. Life provides the opportunities necessary to achieve this goal, but unless one has been made aware by one's mentors that such opportunities abound, one will pass them by, totally unaware of their existence or their significance. Such awareness requires the cultivation of one's powers of observation, plus a critical and dispassionate, yet non-judgmental, recollection of unusual events, chains of circumstance, and encounters with new therapies, both successful and disastrous. It is by our prompt analysis of each new event, procedure, or treatment, that we build a fund of knowledge over the years which constitutes the experience that provides the foundation for the art and science of our medical practice. Not only does it reduce the changes of our making the same error twice, it also gives us the ability, often under adverse circumstances, and frequently with incomplete information, to make correct decisions.

In the cardiac surgical arena, several keys facilitate the conversion of experience to effective action. The first is the indispensability of *constant vigilance*. We are surrounded by assassins at every turn. It is truly amazing how quickly, and with what diabolic persistence, a small piece of adventitia or arteriosclerotic debris will find its way into a coronary arteriotomy and be responsible for a subsequent, unexplained obstruction of that vessel. A suture may become tangled or stuck to a glove and result in the abrupt avulsion of a graft from its newly completed anastomosis. It is equally amazing how focused one's attention can be upon a small part of a small operative field, with great mischief gathering beyond one's immediate field of vision. Operating upon the heart means paying attention at all times to the myriad rhythms of the room—the motion of the lungs, the color of the blood, the flashing of the monitors, the chirping of the alarms, even the sound of suction applied to chest tubes in a partially closed chest varying rhythmically with each heart beat.

The second is the ability to *communicate* to physicians in the same or different disciplines that a problem exists and must be remedied. It is easiest to do this when the problem originates with the patient, rather than when the problem is an error of omission or commission by another physician that unceremoniously upsets your carefully-stacked apple cart. Sometimes, there is nothing worse than being right, as Whistler so eloquently discussed in his treatise, *The Gentle Art of Making Enemies, As Pleasingly Exemplified in Many Instances, Wherein the Serious Ones of this Earth, Carefully Exasperated, Have Been Prettily Spurred on to Unseemliness and Indiscretion, While Overcome by an Undue Sense of Right.*

The third is the wisdom of having a *standardized approach* to cardiac surgical procedures, and the maintenance of *simplicity*. A predictable, orderly sequence of events creates an easy rhythm to which everyone can accommodate and integrate his or her activities. The anesthesiologist should maintain the heart rate and blood pressure within limits to minimize ischemia, and be able to anticipate cannulations, bleedbacks, and manual retraction of the heart. The surgeon, while maintaining the ability to alter the surgical plan, should not change the normal sequence of activities without forewarning, so that every member of the team can readjust and arrive at the same stage of the operation at the same time. It is always awkward to request a clamp and receive a scalpel!

Finally, it is essential that members of the team be able to anticipate the next step in a procedure. This can be done only if the basic order of events has been preserved. It also presupposes that everyone knows the steps to follow in the first place. Any changes in sequence, or introduction of new instrumentation or technology, should be the subject of an in-service training session, or even dry run, until everyone is comfortable with the revised procedure.

We should remember that we are all part of an intimidating, unwelcome, and terrifying experience for most patients who become suddenly aware that their organic integrity is about to be violated, their mortality confronted. Our patients exhibit great courage and trust as they face the unknown at the mercy of strangers who now control events that affect the quality of their lives and even their ultimate survival. As they submit to our ministrations, it is our obligation to maintain vigilance, to open communication between colleagues, to standardize and simplify procedures, and to anticipate outcomes, so that we really are in a position to *lead* our patients, not follow them.

By constantly adding to our fund of knowledge, by recognizing our limitation, and by never hesitating to request assistance when needed, we can reduce the incidence of near misses and spare our patients the devastation of a direct hit—a consummation devoutly to be wished!

Index

entrapment, 107–109
   and femoral artery, 65–66
   perforation, 108
isoproterenol, 10
isoproterenol hydrochloride, 78
isuprel, 10

Judkins approach angiography, 117
jugular vein and cannulation, 132

laparascope, 120
laryngospasm, 68
laser angioplasty, 42
left anterior descending artery
   angioplasty risk, 42
   occlusion and ventricular septal defects, 54
left ventricle. *See also* ventricular fibrillation
   aneurysm, 39–40
   assist device, 28–29, 48
   and cardiopulmonary bypass, 48
   ischemia, 78
   power failure, 36–37
   septal defect, 53–55
Levophed, 73
levothyroxine, 74–75
lidocaine, 74, 116, 123
   and free radical formation, 28

mannitol, 6
Manouguian procedure, 98
mediastinitis, 45–46, 51–52, 120
mediastinum
   hematoma, 111–113
   and peritoneum, air passage, 120
metastatic masses, 67–68
methylprednisolone, 78
mitral valve, 5
   papillary muscles, 54
   rupture versus ventricular septal defect,
differential diagnosis, 54
mitral valve replacement, 24. *see also* prosthetic valve
   and internal thoracic artery graft, 135–137
   and pleural effusion, 131–133
   and thrombosis, 13–15
muscle bridge division, 1–2
muscle relaxants and airway obstruction, 68
myocardial infarction
   and congestive heart failure, 65–66
   and ventricular fibrillation, 115–117
   and ventricular septal defect, 53–55
myocardium, perfusion, 36

needle venting, 6
neurologic injury and air embolism, 6

Nicks procedure, 98
nifedipine, 78
nitroglycerine, 4, 10
nitroprusside, 32
no-reflow phenomenon, 28
norepinephrine bitartate, 73
Nunez procedure, 98

oropharynx and airway obstruction, 68
oxygenator
   and air embolism, 6
   recirculation shunt, clamping, 71–72

pacemaker
   adhesions, 92
   complications, 122–125
   infection, 91–93
   lead perforation of vessels, 123–125
   lead removal, 91–93
   and valve prosthesis, 125
papillary muscle, rupture, 106
pectoral muscle flap rotation, 46
peptic ulcer, mitral insufficiency misdiag-
nosed as, 105–106
perfusionist, 57–58, 71–72, 136
   and anesthesiologist, 72
   and anticoagulants, 72
   and clamping, 72
perfusion pressure and aortic dissection, 2
pericardial tamponade, 19–21, 120, 136
   and aortic dissection, 32, 102
   and biventricular failure, differentiation,
      20
   and central venous cannulation, 133
   and coagulopathy, 128–129
   delayed, 74
   diagnosis, 20
   and pacemaker lead, 124
pericardiocentesis, 124
peripheral vascular disease, 90
peritoneum infection, 119–121
pharmacologic treatment versus cardiopulmonary bypass, 48
phenolanine mesylate, 73
phosphodiesterase inhibitor, 36
pleural effusion, 81–83, 131–133
pneumoperitoneum, 119–121
pneumothorax, tension, 68, 125
porcine bioprosthesis, 97–99
positron emission tomography and akinetic
myocardial segments, 48
potassium
   toxicity, 9–11
   and venous endothelium, 36
pressure transducer, 124

proscoline, 78
prostaglandins, 78
prosthetic valve, 73. *See also* mitral valve
    replacement
    and air embolism, 95–96
    annular abscesses, 52, 99
    and aorto-ventricular discontinuity, 97–99
    biologic versus mechanical, 14, 98
    and infection, 52, 99
    and pacemaker, 125
    structural failure, comparisons, 98
    sutures, 97–99
    thrombosis, 13–15
prostoglandin E_1, 10
protamine, 4, 63
    and heparin, 10
    reaction, 10, 64
protamine sulfate, 78
providone-iodine. *See* Betadine
pulmonary artery
    and aortic dissection, 102
    catheter perforation, 3–4
    hypertension, 77–79
pulmonary edema, 23, 47, 57
    and mitral insufficiency, 105–106
pulmonary hypertension, 77–79
pulomonary hypertension
    and infants, 78

quinidine, 59

radionuclide imaging, 20
radionuclide wall motion study, 48
ranitidine hydrochloride, 78
reoperation, 119–121
    and amiodarone side effects, 59–61
    and defibrillation pads, 135–137
    and infection, 51–52
    and occult hypotension, 73–75
    and potassium toxicity, 9–11
    and sternal division, 135–137
    and sternotomy infection, 31–33, 51–52
retroperfusion, 96
right atrial tamponade, 20
right bundle branch block and pulmonary
    artery catheterization, 4
right coronary artery
    dissection, 115–117
    and septal-apical defects, 54
roto-ablation, 42

St. Jude prosthesis, 13, 14, 98, 106
    and aortic dissection, 102
saline and catheter insertion, 4
saphenous veins, 3

allografts, 86
alternatives, 85–87
lesser, 86
ultrasonic scan check, 87
scrub nurse, 72
simplicity and cardiac surgery, 140
sinogram, 32
sinus bradycardia, 116
sodium bicarbonate, 10
sodium warfarin, 14
Sones approach angiography, 116–117
splenic artery, aneurysm, 90
standardization of approach, 140
Staphylococcus aurea infection, 23, 51–52, 91–93
sternotomy, infection, 31–33, 45–46, 51–52
steroids, 6
ST-segment, 27, 47
    and ventricular fibrillation, 115, 116
sutures
    and aneurysm, 40, 103
    and aortic annulus, 97–99
    and infection, 52
    and mediastinitis, 52
Swan-Ganz catheter, 65, 95
    artery perforation, 3–4
    and subpleural hemorrhage, 83
    and ventricular septal defect diagnosis, 54

teamwork and surgery, xi–xii, 72, 83,
    139–140
Technetium-99m ventriculography, 73
    and pericardial tamponade, differential
    diagnosis, 20
tension pneumothorax, 68, 125
thallium scanning and akinetic myocardial
    segments, 48
thiopental, 6
thoracotomy, 108, 113
thrombolysis, 27
thrombosis, 13–15
thyroid hormones, 74–75
traction and pacemaker lead removal, 92
transesophageal echocardiography, 20
transfusion reaction, 78
transmural infarction, 45
transplant, 28–29, 48
Trendlenburg position, 6, 96
tricuspid valve, 92

ultrasonic scan check of veins, 87
uremia, 74
urine output, impaired, 1, 2

valve prosthesis. *See* prosthetic valve
vena cava